It's not chemo.
It's therapy.

Rob Huthnance

It's not chemo. It's therapy.

Editing and book design by Kelly Andersson

ISBN-10: 0991070291
ISBN-13: 978-0-9910702-9-9

ITSNOTCHEMO.COM

Published in the United States by Charter & Cage Press

13 14 15 16 17 18   10 9 8 7 6 5 4 3 2 1

For Doctors Nokleberg, Oh and Shires

I think EVERYONE at times wonders how they would react after hearing from a doctor that they, or their family member, has the dreaded "C"! Reading Rob's weekly emails about Charlotte's illness and their family's reaction to it not only re-affirmed my admiration for the entire Huthnance family, but also gave me a new optimism that MY reaction to the reality of a serious family illness could indeed be marked by positivity, hope, faith, love and ultimate success.

Many people are able to sift through the emotional baggage of a traumatic experience with the wisdom of hindsight. Rob and Charlotte's ability to handle the emotional baggage of such trauma in "real time" is nothing short of inspiring. And ... dude can write!

~ *recording artist Jack Ingram*

CONTENTS

FOREWORD

It's Not Chemo is an inside look at one family's experience with chemotherapy treatment in the face of ovarian cancer. The book includes a long series of email updates sent by Rob Huthnance to a large circle of friends and family – a circle that grew each week to eventually include hundreds of followers who waited each Friday for the updates on Charlotte's progress. It's a heart-warming story of courage in the face of adversity, cheer and faith in the presence of what could have been gloomy defeat.

The example set by both Charlotte and Rob Huthnance – and all the members of Team Charlotte – will inspire readers to believe in the power of prayer and to try harder to survive challenges beyond conventional expectations. While each of us will always face challenges, the story of Team Charlotte personifies the values and optimistic spirit that have so characterized the American people as a group as we have turned challenges into opportunities in the history of this country.

During my travels across our country and around the world, I have spoken with, listened to, and made friends with people from all walks of life. One common theme I've recognized is people's clarity of purpose in life – which is serving others and doing our best to leave this world better than we found it.

I've witnessed numerous fine examples of "leadership" over the last 30 or so years, and the Huthnance story must be included on the list. Rob Huthnance, as a husband and father, provided leadership to his family, friends, close helpers, and what developed into a huge online community of supporters during Charlotte's treatment. Charlotte herself provided a very different but no less admirable example of leadership with her unwavering trust in the Lord, her determination to not wilt in the face of what to many would seem an insurmountable foe, and her persistent display of "Charlitude" in caring for others and offering cheer and inspiration to those around her.

A tragic need always brings out the realization of our deep dependence on the One who holds our future, and this book details one such story. In many ways, the essential foundation of any relationship is trust – and that is certainly true in the story of Team Charlotte. Rob trusted Charlotte to do her best, to battle through the many weeks of chemotherapy and to hold on to her positive attitude, her faith, and her determination to survive – and survive with the joy that only Christ can provide. At the same time, Charlotte had to trust Rob to maintain the family routine, assume new household responsibilities he was neither familiar with nor good at, and stand loyally by her side. Their children had to trust both parents to keep them in the circle, to be honest with them, and to care for them with some semblance of normalcy in a home life that could very well have dissolved without that parental leadership. The lot of them had to trust their extended family and their close friends to lift them up in prayer and support them through a bewildering short-term future with which they'd had but little experience.

And it worked. Why? Faith. Faith, trust, teamwork and action.

I have often said over the years that rhetoric without results is worthless, and that we as a country and as individuals need deeds, not words. *It's Not Chemo* offers a sterling example of how individuals can work together and act to help others. How many times have you heard, after a family or medical crisis, "Let me know if you need anything" or other similar words? Charlotte's friends did not wait for her to let them know – they identified what she needed and they acted on that. Team Charlotte should be an inspiration for all of us as individuals – and for the groups and communities to which we belong – to act rather than merely ask. It is through our actions that we build the communities in which God intended us to live. The best of the human spirit includes that spark that moves us to action, to help and assist, without being asked.

When we fulfill that part of the human role then we can say, as Rob Huthnance does in his book, "I genuinely tried to do my best."

Donald L. Evans
34th United States Secretary of Commerce

PREFACE

When we learned that my wife Charlotte needed surgery to remove two large and potentially cancerous tumors from her abdomen, I did what a lot of people do these days. I sent an email alerting friends and family about our situation. After Charlotte's surgery, I sent another email update. Toward the end of her hospital stay, I sent another.

During this beginning stage of her excursion with cancer, many people encouraged me to set up a blog or join one of the websites where I could post updates for all to view. These propositions felt uncomfortable. In a world where social media can get out of control, we wanted to control our situation as best we could and decided against these avenues. I took charge of communication by drafting and sending an email every Friday.

The personal touch of the direct email felt natural. We had direct correspondence with our community, and their responses brought smiles to our faces – often in a manner that would have been inappropriate had the responder posted a reply online for the world to read.

What we didn't contemplate or comprehend was the buzz the weekly emails would create and the power of the forward button. Hundreds of people were on the original distribution list; thousands and thousands read the emails.

As the emails were shared again and again, complete strangers became our friends. Each reader, however, had a tie either directly or indirectly to our family, and while we had lost the control we'd originally sought, knowing that someone cared enough to share our story with a circle of friends provided us the motivation to continue.

As the readership grew and our endeavor gained traction, people waited with anticipation on Fridays for the weekly email. They wanted to read the message for themselves and share it immediately. As the emails evolved into more than just medical updates, readers used them for self-inspiration, personal reflection and, believe it or not, even material for Sunday school class.

This buzz and level of anticipation are the foundation for this book. As you read on, visualize this positive energy our community created and breathed for so many months. I suspect our medical story is relatively common, but our journey, attitudes, lessons learned, and community's response are very rare and defining.

All of us involved hope and anticipate that through our story, others' lives can be made better.

INTRODUCTION

We like our cocktails, and we cook with real butter. Otherwise, by all accounts, we have lived healthy lives. We never contemplated the possibility of getting sick at the age of 39. Thank the Lord that Charlotte never missed an annual physical with her doctor.

It's not chemo. It's therapy.

CHAPTER 1
HAVE OUR LIVES JUST CHANGED FOREVER?

From: Rob Huthnance
Date: December 15, 2011 9:51:02 PM CST
To: Rob Huthnance
Subject: Charlotte

Friends,

This email is a prayer request. Nothing more, nothing less. We will gladly provide further information as we learn more, but this is what we know.

Last week Charlotte had her annual doctor's appointment. Her doctor had some concern and suggested that she have an ultrasound and sonogram just for good measure. An appointment was made for Tuesday morning. The tests revealed a mass in her abdomen, and she was immediately called back to the hospital for a CT scan. It showed a mass consistent with ovarian cancer.

This afternoon we met with a gynecologic oncologist. By reputation, he is the best there is. We liked him a lot; moreover, you could just tell he is extremely good at what he does.

She has two tumors. One is the size of a grapefruit on her ovary, and the other is the size of an apple in her abdomen next to her large intestine. Surgery is scheduled for Tuesday, and pathology testing will be performed during the operation. Once we have the pathology report, the doctor will know how to proceed with the surgery.

IF, repeat IF, in fact the tumors are cancerous, he will be as aggressive as possible during surgery. Regarding ovarian cancer, long-term success is directly tied to the initial surgery. We want him to get it all. Period.

We are encouraged that we have a solid plan and an all-star team of doctors. Unfortunately, there are a lot of unknowns that will exist until the surgery.

Our family is very supportive, and we are well covered regarding food and activities.

Please feel free to forward this email to anyone you believe will send a couple of prayers our way.

Thank you.

Rob

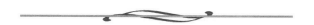

Charlotte's annual doctor's appointment was Wednesday, December 7th. It was a routine doctor's appointment that had been scheduled twelve months in advance at her appointment the year before. Since we had no concern about the appointment, I thought nothing of going to Houston that morning for business. The plan was for Charlotte to join me the next day for a company Christmas party Thursday night. She would fly back to Dallas on Friday, and I would drive with my brother, who lives in Houston, to our family's ranch for the weekend.

When she and I spoke on the phone Wednesday night, I could tell something was awry, but she didn't express the severity of concern her doctor had regarding the mass she felt in her abdomen. Charlotte flew in midday on Thursday. Late that afternoon before the party, we discussed her need to have further testing, but she carried her nerves well so I had zero apprehension. The party that night was fun. There were lots of cocktails, a little tomfoolery, and a hysterical white elephant gift exchange. Friday morning I dropped her off at the airport, and she flew back to Dallas. I had a fun weekend at the ranch with guys, and because of Charlotte's demeanor, I had no reason to fret over the weekend. When I arrived at home Sunday afternoon, all seemed normal. I simply dealt with the standard issues of re-entry to the family after a weekend away.

At 8 a.m. Tuesday, we arrived at the hospital for her sonogram. She checked in, we read the newspaper in the waiting room, she was called back, I waited some more. Then we gathered our things and went home. It was no big deal. They told us they would get back to us in the next day or so. The home phone rang at 10:45 a.m. The person on the other end of the line said the sonogram showed a mass, and we needed to come back to the hospital as quickly as possible to have a CT scan. The radiologist "squeezed" us in for an appointment at 1 p.m.

After checking in, we were escorted to the back of the office and were shown some chairs in which to wait. Charlotte went into a little room next door and drank "the stuff." As we were waiting for the stuff to illuminate her insides, reality was starting to kick in – we wouldn't be back at the hospital this quickly if this weren't serious. Our faces were solemn, and I'm sure we looked scared. We could hardly look at each other much less make small talk. About this time another couple sat down next to us. A few minutes later the woman stood up, walked over to Charlotte and whispered, "I'd like to give you a hug." Charlotte looked at her, a little puzzled. Then in the soothing, reassuring manner of chosen, wise, African American women, she said, "It looks like you got bad news today. I got bad news today as well. I'd like to give you hug so that you know it's going to be okay." I'm convinced this incredible person had wings – even if just for this moment. We sensed the presence of the Lord and felt peaceful about the future.

We were sent home after her scan around 3:30 – and before 5 o'clock, the phone rang. It was Charlotte's gynecologist, and she said she had discussed the CT scan with the radiologist. There was a mass in her abdomen that had to be removed, and while they didn't know for sure, it did show all the signs of ovarian cancer. Her doctor had already scheduled an appointment for us on Thursday with the gynecological oncologist that she recommended.

We both love Charlotte's gynecologist. She delivered two of our three children, is our age, lives in our neighborhood, and has children in school with ours. We trusted her. Whatever she said went.

All day Wednesday, before the appointment on Thursday, we fretted and called our doctor friends to check up on the oncologist whom we had no reason to know. Miraculously, but not surprisingly, we only heard incredible reports about his abilities and reputation. My parents are friends with a person who happens to be a world-renowned surgeon in Dallas, and my mother called him to inquire about our new doctor. His response was that the oncologist was one of the best in his field. Then he paused and declared, "No, he is the best in his field." The best was now officially Charlotte's oncologist.

During the consultation on Thursday the doctor discussed the imminent surgery and what would take place. He discussed the hospital stay required, the probability of time in intensive care, and what would happen if the tumors turned out to be cancerous. He was very deliberate and calming. I, of course, asked too many questions, and after a series of them, he looked at Charlotte and could tell she'd had enough. He said he didn't think she wanted to hear all of these questions and answers, and he was right. He wrangled me in perfectly, and I stopped talking. After listening to him, we felt assured that he would do everything in his power during surgery to promote long-term success. We left his office and drove toward home thinking, "I can't … believe … this is real."

Thursday we had a couple of close friends over to the house. We just sat around the den in bewilderment. The sentiment was that I needed to send our friends and family an email alerting everyone about what was happening. A couple of glasses of wine later (and maybe a glass of scotch, too), the above email hit the wire and our world forever changed.

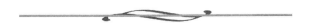

That weekend was the longest and yet shortest four-day weekend of all time. Between the appointment with the oncologist on Thursday and the surgery on Tuesday, things were pretty hectic. However, the craziness was welcomed because I turned numb every time I was alone, and I was about out of adrenaline. I took an Ambien every night just so I could sleep three or four hours.

In an effort to promote a positive attitude and reduce negative energy, Charlotte did not want to be around tears. There were plenty of tears behind closed doors, and that was enough. Therefore, when she saw friends, she wanted those moments to be upbeat. To illustrate this, a girlfriend who is very funny by nature came over as soon as she heard the news. Not knowing what to do or say, with tears in her eyes, she simply gave Charlotte a huge hug. After the hug, Charlotte looked at her and said,

"Okay, you have to stop crying. Go outside and compose yourself and then come back in. If you can't, that's okay, but you will have to leave and come back later. We are not having sad moments around here." The girlfriend respected Charlotte's wishes, collected herself, and then made everyone at the house laugh with her usual wit and hilarity. Her sense of humor is so palpable that at times it's frustrating because you genuinely wish you were as consistently on your game as she is.

On Friday, Charlotte and I gathered the children together. We have three – one boy (Thompson, in third grade) and two girls (C.C. in first grade and Georgeann who is Pre-K). We were aware of the drama that could be created, and we were scared that we would scare them. We didn't want to mention cancer. We didn't know – truly. We told them that Mommy had a bump in her belly, and the doctor needed to take it out. That was the truth. My son, like so many first-born children, is wise beyond his years. A little boy across the street had been diagnosed with a rare form of cancer two years before. My children were very well versed about cancer because of their friendship with the boy across the street. Thompson asked, "Is it cancer?"

From moment one, we had decided that it would be easier to tell the truth to the children. If we gave only true information, then we wouldn't have to keep up with what we could and couldn't say. We might not volunteer everything, but if they asked, we would talk openly about it. He asked. So I answered, "It might be. We won't know until after the doctor removes whatever it is that is growing inside her." This seemed to make sense to them and wasn't overly scary, and there were no more questions, so we simply went on about our business.

While many friends and family lived the next few days hoping and claiming and knowing that the tumors were benign, I somehow found solace in the doctors' opinion that it was ovarian cancer. I was very hopeful that they were wrong, of course, but their candor gave me a few days to get my arms around what was to come. I found that the prospect of her having cancer truly helped me prepare myself mentally and emotionally.

CHAPTER 2
THE CANCER IS REAL

From: Rob Huthnance
Date: December 20, 2011 2:54:01 PM CST
To: Rob Huthnance
Subject: Charlotte

Dear Team Charlotte,

Charlotte did very well throughout her surgery. She is now
resting comfortably in her room — a regular room, not intensive
care.

Unfortunately, we did get the news the doctors told us to expect.
She has ovarian cancer, but the doctor was able to remove 100
percent of the disease during surgery.

We were expecting the surgery to take between 2½ and 6 hours,
and they finished in just under 3 hours. In order to remove all of
the cancer, the doctor had to remove her uterus, both ovaries,
part of her colon, and part of her intestine. They were able to
reconnect her entire bowel tract, and her system should be fully
functional in due time. We are very happy that she did not
require a colostomy, and she did not require a blood transfusion.

We believe she will be in the hospital for approximately a week —
a little longer than we had hoped, but clearly this is the best
place for her to begin the recovery process. She will need to gain
her strength back as quickly as possible so that she can
effectively absorb the chemotherapy treatments that are
forthcoming in the near future. To that end, please understand
that we really want to limit visitor traffic. She needs to take
advantage of her time in the hospital.

It's not chemo. It's therapy.

All of you know the feeling when you accomplish a required task to the absolute best of your ability. It feels incredible, and there's no other feeling like it. Think of the adrenaline. Think of the satisfaction. Think of the subsequent pep in your step. Dr. Oh nailed the surgery, he had these feelings, and it was an outright pleasure to watch his natural high as he discussed it afterward.

Thank you all so much for the love, support, and prayers. Every prayer was heard, and all of the love has been felt.

I promise to stay in touch.

Rob

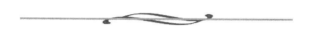

I love watching people do their best, especially if they are good at what they do, whether it's Josh Hamilton hitting four home runs in one game, a businessman with a Midas touch, a child who innately comprehends the 88 keys of the piano, or in this case a doctor saving someone's life. It's just cool. Really cool.

We arrived at the hospital at 5 a.m. It felt like a duck hunt, only the lack of sleep the night before didn't come from too many funny stories and hearing someone around the campfire howl, "Come on … just one more drink." I didn't sleep for obvious reasons.

My parents were in town and Charlotte's best friend from college also came. Charlotte's parents and brothers got to the hospital shortly after we did. Around 6 a.m., several doctor friends who were on call stopped by our pre-op room. I would not have thought about this previously, but having these doctors swing by to say hello was very comforting and meaningful. Charlotte was wheeled away around 7 a.m., and the rest of us were resigned to hanging out in the waiting room for a few hours.

When I walked into the waiting room, there were already friends there. I couldn't believe it. It was almost like a surprise party. Then as the clock ticked on, more and more people showed up. My little brother and sister-in-law surprised me with their presence around 8:15. They had rearranged work schedules and children's events and caught the first flight from Houston. They were a sight for sore eyes. Everyone's attendance was such a tribute to Charlotte. There were easily four times as many friends as there were seats in the waiting room. There was one other family in there, and I genuinely felt sorry for them, as they were totally overwhelmed. One of my friends brought a game of Scrabble. As dorky as it sounds, it was pure genius. We played without a clock so I could have the liberty to speak with people as they wandered by my little corner. I highly suggest Scrabble (or something like it) in the waiting room. It gives the participants something to do where they actually have to use their brains, yet it is brainless at the same time. It was a great way to pass the time.

I don't think the doctor had ever seen so many people in the waiting room during one of his surgeries. I think he was more than taken aback. After being directed my way by a few people, he and I made eye contact, and I jumped up and followed him down the hall. My parents and Charlotte's parents followed us into a small room. He said the surgery was very successful but that the mass was malignant. He told us everything that he had removed, and he said she would be in post-op for a little while. While numb, none of us in the room seemed shocked. We all absorbed the body blow, caught our breath, and regained our composure.

I left the little room with the burden of telling everyone anxiously waiting down the hall. I felt prepared for this, but I don't think anyone else was. They hadn't heard what I had heard in the doctors' voices.

I was determined not to cry while delivering the most poignant speech of my life. During the twenty-yard walk back to the waiting room, I had dozens of eyes focused on me waiting for me to stop and talk. I simply repeated what the doctor had told us. The surgery went well, but it was cancer. Instantly, the hopeful faces fell to frowns, and the tears welled up in our friends' eyes. It was difficult to make eye contact with everyone.

As part of the post-surgery routine, the doctors and nurses want the patient to be awake, even if just for a minute here and there. The anesthesia medication really makes your mouth and lips dry, and the first time Charlotte came to all she could do was beg for some Chapstick. One of the most helpful people throughout Charlotte's time fighting cancer took on this challenge and sprinted to the gift shop. Having no idea which brand or flavor Charlotte wanted, she simply bought one of each, or 14 to be exact. It was awesome. The bag full of Chapstick lightened the room and was the right thing to do. If given the same assignment, I would have stared at all the choices for several minutes trying to figure out the right one to purchase. I would have compared brands, flavors, and prices. However, after witnessing her "buy them all" technique, here's what I learned – just spend the extra $6 and buy them all.

The day of the surgery we placed each of our children with friends for the day. These friends were very nice about keeping them, and volunteered that our children could even spend the night. I politely declined the invitation because I needed to tell the children what was going on. I didn't want them to hear from someone else that their mother had cancer.

I asked that each of the children be home by 6 p.m. so we could have a family meeting. Everyone understood and obliged. One mom did leave the offer open for C.C. to return to their house if she felt like it after our little meeting.

I gathered everyone in the living room, and we all sat on the couch. Trying to stay true to our commitment of being truthful with them, I told them about the day. With as much calm as my voice could convey, I told them that the doctor found cancer in Mommy's tummy, but he was able to cut it all out. My son was so relieved to hear that the doctor was able to remove all of the cancer. My middle daughter wanted to know what color the cancer was, and my youngest simply gazed at me with her big brown eyes.

After a few minutes of light conversation, they felt good about the report and were ready to do something else. Thompson played video games, C.C. wanted to go back to her friend's house, and Georgeann colored in a coloring book with her grandmother. There was no hype or drama, and everybody seemed okay.

We took turns spending the night on the couch in the hospital room. I was very grateful that Charlotte's mother and friends were willing to help me with this duty. It wasn't fun, and there was effectively no sleeping involved with all of the beeping equipment and nurse activity.

Spending a week in the hospital provides the family a lot of idle time. I can tell you about every nook and cranny in the wing of the hospital, which icemaker worked the best and which pot of coffee was the least bad. By way of good fortune, a brand-new 40,000 square foot liquor store, one block from the hospital, opened for business that week. I spent an hour inside it at a time, and I visited the store several times. The store even had a deli. There were twenty sandwiches on the menu, and I think I tried seven of them.

A long-time friend of mine is a doctor, and we spoke often during the hospital stay. During one of our visits, he professed how the community was going to hold us up and together. I mention this later in one of the updates. The community support sounded special and was something I wanted to hear; however, I had no idea what that really meant. The salutation to start this week's email changed from "Friends" to "Team Charlotte." Clearly this Team had been formed and was coming together.

It's not chemo. It's therapy.

CHAPTER 3
COMPLETELY EXHAUSTED AND TOTALLY NUMB

From: Rob Huthnance
Date: December 29, 2011 6:12:15 PM CST
To: Rob Huthnance
Subject: 12/29/11 Update for Charlotte

Dear Team Charlotte,

Charlotte came home Monday afternoon. The children and I are very pleased to have her home, and she has enjoyed sleeping in her own bed. She is still sore but is recovering on schedule.

We met with the oncologist today to discuss chemotherapy options and next steps. Thankfully, there are not a lot of options for us to wade through and choose. The two drugs used during chemotherapy have been used to treat ovarian cancer for twenty years. The drugs are even available generically.

Microscopic cancer cells are very likely still present. They are aggressive and need to be treated immediately. Starting chemo treatments as soon as possible is imperative; therefore, her first session will be on Thursday, January 5th.

Her chemotherapy treatments will be administered weekly for the next eighteen weeks. They will be given at the oncologist's office via IV.

Thank you to all for the unbelievable amount of support. We don't know how her body will respond to chemo, and we don't know what will trigger the obvious emotions. Please be patient with us as we work to understand the new normal. This includes meals, visits, laughter sessions, crying sessions, angry sessions, grateful sessions, chemo friends, carpool, babysitting, and end-of-the-day wine sessions — yes the doctor said it was okay.

Charlotte has her age, strength, faith, and support on her side. She's ready to win.

Rob.

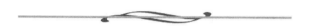

I just went through the motions to get this update out. I was tired, I'd spent a week at the hospital, my wife was tired and sore from surgery, my children were ready to have their mother back, I was nervous about chemotherapy and how we would manage a family with our quarterback at half strength, and I had close friends saying I needed to send something out. So I sent the email.

All that we could think about was the impending chemotherapy. Have you ever heard of a good chemotherapy experience? We hadn't either. The anxiety was off the charts. The only thing I could imagine was a miserable Saturday morning hangover in college. There is a reason no one drinks trashcan punch past the age of 21.

Candidly, I was relieved that I wouldn't be the one hugging the toilet, but I really didn't want to take on all the responsibilities of the healthy person either. I envisioned a lot to coordinate, and it made my head hurt. I know that's lousy to say, but it's the truth. There's a lot of stress that hits the caretaker at this point in the process. There are so many unknowns, and these unknowns really beat you down.

What I failed to mention in the update was our Christmas before Charlotte came home. We were bound and determined to make Christmas as normal as we could for our children. My parents were staying at our house, and we took care of everything. Santa Claus came as advertised, and we all had fun playing with the new toys and emptying our stockings. After the newness wore off, we had some breakfast, my father showered and donned his red cardigan sweater that comes out only at Christmas, for the last forty-one Christmases.

Next we gathered around the Christmas tree to open our presents. We separated Charlotte's into her own pile. Surprisingly, the children never missed a beat. They knew their mother was doing well, and they were thrilled with all of the new stuff. After the presents were opened, I set the table as close as I could to how Charlotte would have done it. I think I got it about 85 percent there, red tablecloth, Christmas linen napkins, fine china, silverware, crystal and all. I took a picture and sent it to Charlotte at the hospital. She was very appreciative of the effort and was surprised that we had done so much.

Charlotte's parents spent most of the day with her at the hospital, and we took the children up there around 6 p.m. We brought her a couple of the presents we had set aside earlier, and everyone had fun with our non-traditional Christmas. My parents took the children home, and I stayed with Charlotte a few more hours.

This week Team 18 was created. It was the most incredible idea. Knowing daily errands and tasks would be the last thing Charlotte would want to do during her 18-week chemotherapy stint, her friends each took a week, starting this week, and became Charlotte's personal assistant. They went grocery shopping, ran errands, went to the pharmacy and generally did anything, I mean anything, Charlotte asked. This is such a brilliant and fairly easy way to truly help. These women were going to the grocery store every couple days anyway to support their own families. Why couldn't they pick up an extra bottle of Tide, a gallon of milk, or whatever other item our house was low on? It required minimal effort and lifted such a burden.

The process they set up was pretty savvy, too. On Monday morning, the team member responsible for the week would text Charlotte asking how she could help. Charlotte would text back a couple of items or to-dos. Then once they were completed, the team member would text Charlotte letting her know the items were on the porch. No one had to spend any energy or have any awkward moments on the phone or in person. All apprehension and pressure were removed from the situation.

What this group of women didn't know or contemplate at the time was how much this was going to promote Charlotte's healing. They simply thought they were being helpful. Charlotte recovered from surgery so quickly and so completely because she did not have to spend energy going to the grocery store or running errands. She could focus all her energy into healing and being with her family.

CHAPTER 4
GAME ON – LET'S WIN

From: Rob Huthnance
Date: January 6, 2012 5:51:27 PM CST
To: Rob Huthnance
Subject: 1/6/12 Charlotte Update

Dear Team Charlotte,

The first round of chemo has officially come and gone, and she is doing remarkably well.

Thank you for all the kind words I have received regarding the email updates. I have found these brief messages to be very cathartic. I really wanted to choose a different, more common word than "cathartic" because Charlotte is going to make fun of me for using it; however, it's the only word that truly fits. My definition of the word is a release of emotional tension and, consequently, spiritual renewal. Thank you for allowing me this opportunity for free therapy.

My goal is to provide everyone an update on Fridays. Some weeks this email may be sent out Thursday night, and some weeks it may be Saturday morning. Because you all are friends, you probably recall that I have been known to have an occasional affair with the 19th hole on Friday afternoons … nevertheless, as chemo treatments will be on Thursdays, Fridays are my goal.

As she does with most things in life, Charlotte decided to be proactive regarding her cancer. She decided in the hospital bed while recovering from surgery that she was going to cut off her hair and donate it to Locks of Love, an organization that makes wigs for those in need. As advertised, on Tuesday she went to the hair salon and had over twelve inches of hair cut off and sent to the foundation. Had I known how good she was going to look with super short hair, I would have encouraged her to cut it off years ago. She looks great.

We checked into the "infusion suite" at the doctor's office yesterday morning with no idea what to expect. Everyone was very nice and made her feel very comfortable. Of course, she was smiling and making friends with all the nurses.

By the way, yesterday was nurse Janet's 32nd wedding anniversary as she was married in 1980 (this should make the math easy on her husband), and her youngest daughter is 19 and is enjoying college. I mean really? Keep in mind this is in the stinking chemo room ... the only "friend" I made was when another guy whose wife was receiving treatment came up and asked me, "First time here? You can always tell the new guys."

Charlotte received some anti-nausea medicine prior to the chemo medicine. She had no dramatic sickness and took it like a champ for three hours. The most notable side effect so far has been some minor neuropathy in her feet, which means they feel tingly like they are asleep. We aren't naïve enough to think that subsequent rounds won't be more challenging, but so far so good.

There's no doubt in my mind that the forty guys who put themselves, in her honor yesterday, through the hardest CrossFit workout ever conceived must have absorbed a lot of her pain. There's no doubt in my mind that all of the fabulous meals that have been delivered nourished her body to the necessary strength.

There's no doubt in my mind that our smiles are bigger because I have a friend whose only communication with me is a daily phone call that involves no hellos or goodbyes — just a solid joke. And there's no doubt in my mind that the thousands of prayers are working.

Talk to you next week.

Rob

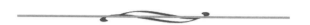

We had no idea what to expect regarding chemotherapy. My father went through it almost twenty years ago, and I don't recall that it was a pleasant experience. I don't recall anyone having a pleasant experience. To my knowledge no one has ever said, "Woo hoo! I get to have chemotherapy today!" We kept waiting for some big sickness event – like a pregnant woman who feels great one minute and throws up in the parking lot the next minute. However, Charlotte felt okay. This made recovery from her surgery a little easier, and we had the strength and energy to tackle another week.

Our appointment for the first chemotherapy session was at 10:30 a.m. on a Thursday. We asked a few friends to pray for us and send some good vibes our way at appointment time that morning. At some point our son caught wind of these requests. He set the alarm on his digital watch for 10:30 a.m. He attends the public elementary school in our neighborhood, and when his alarm went off in the middle of class, unprompted and uncoached, he slid off his chair, knelt on the floor and said a prayer for his mother. He's in third grade and had the moxie to pull this off. None of his friends even thought about teasing him, and the teacher called Charlotte and relayed the story as soon as school was out.

I turned 40 on January 2nd. For years Charlotte had talked about throwing me a 40th birthday party, and she had one in the works before she got sick. The plans changed slightly, but she still pulled it off and attended it for a couple of hours before her bed called her home.

I didn't mention this party in the update because I didn't want to upset anyone who wasn't invited. Charlotte invited twenty-five couples, which is a very challenging size to get the mix right. She did a good job of blending old friends and newer friends, and given the high levels of complaints regarding hangovers the next day, I'm confident that everyone had a blast.

We have been hosting parties on all levels for a long time. Without fail approximately 25 percent of the guest list simply won't be able to attend. There is no doubt that as more of a tribute to Charlotte than to me (feel free to ask around about this), twenty-four of the twenty-five couples showed up. The only couple who didn't make it happened to be on a legitimate business trip – in Hawaii no less.

I could have done a better job describing Charlotte's first encounter with the nurses. She has never met a stranger, and every person she meets likes her. Here we are, surrounded by many sick, not very happy people, and Charlotte is chatting up the nurses with a big smile on her face. Of course, she is so vibrant that the nurses visit with her like they are old friends. One of the nurses goes into all these details about her husband, her children, and her anniversary. This was nice because it did make the time go faster. Meanwhile, I was sitting at a table next to her sterile lounge chair covered with vinyl hoping no one in the room talked to me. I struggle at times finding the enjoyment of making small talk with strangers. I love meeting new people and discussing common things, but I didn't necessarily want to make new friends in the infusion suite. So when the guy called me out for being the new guy, I got a kick out of it.

On the drive home, we were amazed at how well she felt. On the drive up there, we thought she would need a barf bag for the drive home.

We have several friends who have gotten into CrossFit, a workout regimen at franchised gyms that is very strenuous and does not use modern technology. They often ask, "How did the cavemen get strong and fast?" Each of these friends has gone through a transformation of sorts. Clearly their bodies have changed as they are in better shape than they were during off-season football in high school, but their minds have changed as well. The CrossFit community is powerful, and those who have joined can't imagine their life without it. Those of us who don't enjoy super intense workouts at 5 a.m. will never understand. But that's okay – good for them and good for us.

One of my long-time friends who fits the CrossFit mold exactly as described above organized a workout in honor of Charlotte. It was scheduled for Charlotte's first day of chemotherapy. He coerced forty CrossFit friends and brethren to participate in the workout. The WOD (workout of the day), as they call it, was brutal, so much so that he did not detail it on the invitation email. He wanted people to show up. The WOD was affectionately named "Tough Girl," which describes Charlotte's demeanor toward cancer, and was the phrase inscribed on the first pink and white bracelets another friend had made for Charlotte (and Team) right after surgery.

The premise behind the workout was no matter how hard they pushed themselves, it couldn't be as bad as chemotherapy. They were determined to absorb some of her pain through creating their own. No doubt it worked.

One of the easiest questions for friends to ask patients and direct caregivers is "Will you please let me know what I can do to help? I'll do anything." Because it is easy to ask, it is the question most often asked. Unfortunately, it's not easy for anyone hearing that question to answer it. The perceived guilt that comes with answering it can be unbearable and not worth the effort. Can you imagine really asking someone to pick up your dry cleaning? How about asking someone to get you some toothpaste? What about toilet paper? I need my shoes resoled, would you please take them to the shop? It just doesn't happen. So if you really want to help someone, take the burden of asking for help away from the patient and caregiver. Make direct statements and ask direct questions. "I'm going to be running errands all over town tomorrow. Do you need me to pick up your dry cleaning while I'm out? I have to go to the pharmacy and the grocery store. Do you need me to pick up any prescriptions? Do you have enough milk, laundry detergent, and toilet paper?" The question you ask can and should put the patient at ease. It should not cause anxiety as the caregiver debates mentally whether it's really okay to ask for a little help.

Also this week, an old friend from college called and left me a two-minute voicemail. This friend is the youngest of five boys, so you can only imagine how crazy his house was growing up. Not including the fourth brother, he is arguably the funniest person I know (jab intended – he so wants to be the funniest). His stories are endless, and I have entertained hundreds of people over the years with his antics. The stories get a laugh every time I tell one, but no one laughs as hard as I do when I get to hear him tell one that I witnessed in person or have heard numerous times.

He lives in Austin now, and on his voicemail he apologized for not being able to do more for us because he lives in a different city. Then he said that every day at

5 p.m. during Charlotte's chemotherapy he was going to call and tell me a joke. There would be no hellos or goodbyes. He lived up to his promise, called daily, told the joke, threw out the punchline and hung up the phone. It was genius. There was no forced small talk, and I laughed every time, often all by myself in my office. If you are truly funny, this is an incredible gift to give someone who needs a laugh.

The daily jokes gave Charlotte and me something to talk about when I got home. We didn't have to ask each other how our day was. I knew hers wasn't great, and she knew the stress I had at work. The jokes allowed us to start our re-entry conversation with laughter. She always asked what the joke was as soon as I got home. At the time we didn't realize how powerful that was, but not having to talk cancer or even think cancer for a bit was a real blessing. Charlotte and I genuinely love to laugh.

CHAPTER 5
HERE COMES OUR COMMUNITY

From: Rob Huthnance
Date: January 13, 2012 4:15:55 PM CST
To: Rob Huthnance
Subject: 1/13/12 Charlotte Update

Dear Team Charlotte,

This week was a good week. We are thankful and grateful for many things.

I visited with several close friends this week. During one of the conversations, I had the following revelation: If you exclude the fact that cancer really stinks, Charlotte's (our) situation really is pretty good.

Here are the facts. Surgery was a complete success. There is only one viable chemotherapy treatment; therefore, we haven't had to stress over and worry about which option to choose. Other than fatigue, chemotherapy has not had any drastic adverse effects — primarily no nausea or vomiting. She is very mobile and is in good spirits. I believe it is safe to say that when compared with others with cancer, she is in the 95+ percentile. We'll take that all day. We all know several stories of people with significant struggles. We are grateful for our story.

As we have settled into our new routine and lifestyle, we have had many opportunities for praise and thanks. Charlotte had several activities this week including church, Sunday brunch, a mile-and-a-half walk on the treadmill, and an excursion to the mall. We are thankful for each of these events.

It's not chemo. It's therapy.

Three weeks ago, I anticipated that by now the newness of our situation would have worn off and our friends would have drifted back into their routines. I thought with the kids being back in school and the excitement of the new year, we would be left to fend for ourselves. When thinking about that, I didn't have any bitterness; I just figured it was reality. Boy, did I miss on that prediction. If anything, the support has intensified.

The support is coming from so many different angles, too. Everyone can get their mind around meals and carpools, but there is so much more than that going on behind the scenes. People are helping with grocery shopping, car washes, books, magazines, and sweets. There's an endless stream of encouraging notes and emails, the prayers, the bracelets (we have given out more than 600 and reordered more), the smiley face buttons, the smiley face yard art, day visits from out-of-towners, frame-able letters to Charlotte from famous people, manicures at the house, and of course, the daily jokes.

Smiley faces have become a big theme around our house. Thirty days ago I had no idea how cool smiley faces were. They are very cool, and I am grateful every time I see one.

Think of Charlotte the next time you see a bright yellow smiley face and be grateful that she is doing well.

Talk to you next week.

Rob

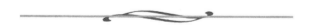

This week we became much more accepting of our situation. It wasn't as frightening as it had been during the previous weeks. We were able to envision what the medical portion of life would be like for the next few months, and with that clarity came comfort and relief. The overall health concerns still existed and were very scary, but the unknowns of chemotherapy were diminished.

We obviously had many worries about the future from the beginning; however, a worry that was ever-present was what life would be like once all our friends went back to their own lives? We should be fine, we thought – they weren't in our lives minutely before cancer and we did fine then, but the attention felt good and was uplifting. We didn't want the support to evaporate overnight.

Friends were so generous with their offers to bring meals for our family. One of Charlotte's friends set up and managed a meal calendar for us. We knew with most meals brought to the house there would be some leftovers; therefore, we limited meals to Mondays and Thursdays. We also knew there would be times when a change of pace would be nice, whether that meant we felt like cooking or maybe going out to eat. Frustratingly for some, but fortunately for us, the meal calendar filled up quickly. I received several calls from people saying "I can't believe the calendar is so full that we can't bring you food until the end of April!?"

A full meal calendar meant there was one less thing we had to think or worry about, and we were very grateful for one less stress in our lives.

People were coming up with things that we never contemplated, things that were so appreciated. One friend sent over a crew to wash our cars. Who doesn't appreciate a clean car? Another friend had a local manicurist swing by the house after work to do Charlotte's toes and fingernails. Charlotte loved this. One girlfriend came over and cleaned out Charlotte's closet, and another girlfriend, an interior designer, helped hang the children's framed artwork in the playroom. Our handyman gave us a day of free service and fixed several items around the house. People consistently gave "their gift." Whatever they were good at, they gave it to us. It was very humbling to watch people contribute their gifts to our situation. Again, I love watching people do what they do best.

The smiley faces first presented themselves in this update. When Charlotte's big brother learned of her probable diagnosis, before the surgery, he went to the store to get her something that would bring a smile to her face. At the store, he had no idea what he was going to purchase. He stumbled across a one-inch yellow smiley face button. He thought it might be fun for her to wear, so he bought it. It was an instant hit the moment he gave it to her. She loved it and had him order 100 more online, and in no time, family and friends were wearing smiley face buttons. Soon thereafter, the nurses and doctors were wearing them at the hospital, and later at the various doctors' offices.

Regarding the smiley faces, the week before, the day of the first chemotherapy session, after spending the morning in the infusion suite, we became electrified when we pulled into our driveway and spotted a dozen smiley faces cut out from bright yellow poster board. They were stapled to wooden stakes and stuck in the ground all over our yard. One of the members of Team 18 had a little fun while we were out, and the only reason she got caught was that she drove back by the scene of the crime one too many times. This started another smiley face epidemic where people throughout the neighborhood placed poster board smiley faces on their front doors or in their front windows. It's amazing how visible a yellow smiley face is from the street.

Sometime around this second week of chemotherapy, a girlfriend of Charlotte's had the idea to order a roll of smiley face stickers. Within a week she had to order several more rolls of stickers. From the beginning, we had a crate on the front porch that held bracelets for anyone who wanted to stop by and grab one. We quickly added stickers to the crate. Supporters were placing these stickers on their back windshields, and hundreds of cars in our neighborhood had bright yellow smiley faces stuck on them. I can't tell you how many I would see driving down the street or in the grocery store parking lot – mostly on cars I didn't recognize. It became a little like a middle school craze, to be cool you had to have sticker on your car. I smiled every time I saw one, and I still do.

Next to the crate of stickers and bracelets we had two more important items. One was a regular sized Igloo cooler, and the other was a whiteboard with a couple of markers beside it. The cooler served as the holding tank for anything and everything – meals, medicine, magazines – you name it. If it was to be picked up from our house or dropped off at our house, it went in the cooler. This eliminated the inevitable chaos and extra time needed for live exchanges at the front door – or the inconvenience of answering the door if you're in your pajamas or in the bathroom.

I wish I could remember who came up with the whiteboard idea because I would like to thank them again. Friends used the whiteboard to leave short, quirky notes. As they drove by the house, it was easy to hop out of the car, run to the porch, write a quick line or two, and drive away. Lots of kids liked writing their names on it as well. It was just a little something that was always happy. It was a gentle reminder that someone was thinking about us.

CHAPTER 6
THANK YOU

From: Rob Huthnance
Date: January 20, 2012 1:59:12 PM CST
To: Rob Huthnance
Subject: 1/20/12 Charlotte Update

Dear Team Charlotte,

We finally feel like we are in a regular routine. We understand the chemo drill, I now better understand how to get the kids fed and off to school, we understand Charlotte's need for extra sleep, and I believe I have found a good balance between work and life.

Other than starting yesterday's treatment 90 minutes after her set appointment, the session went off without a hitch. She got a comfortable spot tucked away where she didn't have to pay much attention to the action in the infusion suite, and the needle was properly located on the first try. Before the big drugs are administered, she receives a dose of anti-nausea medicine as well as some Benadryl. The Benadryl evidently hit the spot because she was able to take a real nap during the treatment. For the rest of the day, her energy level was strong, and she did not feel nauseated or have any tingling in her feet. Three treatments are now in the books.

I have a friend who says only "Thank you" and never "Thanks." Whether it's in person, on the phone, through a text or email, it's always "Thank you." I noticed this some time ago but never confronted him about it. This week I asked. I wanted to know if he made a conscious effort to say "Thank you." His reply was yes, "It's always Thank you, never Thanks." I learned this week that there is a difference between the two.

We make a genuine effort in our home to use our manners and to provide a pleasant atmosphere for our children. Sometimes that means we have to firmly remind family members that just because we are related does not mean we can leave off a "Thank you." However, "Thanks" would normally suffice.

Earlier this week while Charlotte and I were getting ready for bed, she looked at me and said "Thank you" (not "Thanks"). I asked, "For what?" and she said, "Just thank you." It was a nice moment. The next morning I said, "Thank you for saying thank you." It was great. We've been married a long time, and I don't recall our thanking each other.

So over the next couple of days, I decided to experiment with "Thank you" and not my typical, often flippant "Thanks." My first opportunity was at lunch when the bus boy filled my glass of water. I looked him in the eye and said, "Thank you." His face lit up with a smile that was as genuine as I have seen. The "Thank you" opportunities continued. The mailman, the guy at the gas station, the different colleagues at multiple business meetings, and the guy that put extra sauce on my barbecue sandwich at Angelo's yesterday all had the same electric reaction to an honest "Thank you."

We went out for Mexican food Wednesday night. After we finished and were walking back to the car, we noticed that someone had backed into our bumper. You can probably guess what my reaction was. Charlotte quickly found the nice note the gentleman had left on our windshield, and without missing a beat, she said, "Well, it looks like I get to add another person to my team." She called the phone number and left a message. Within twenty minutes the nice man called back and said, "You said 'Thank you' three times on my voicemail. I had to call and visit with you." Next thing you know, they figured out that their families know each other and that Charlotte used to babysit his nieces when we lived in San Antonio. He is now on Team Charlotte.

I don't know why there is a tangible difference between "Thank you" and "Thanks." But there is. It's real. The person receiving the "Thank you" is affected more positively.

Of all the smiles that were created this week following the words "Thank you," none was bigger than mine.

Thank you Team Charlotte. Talk to you next week.

Rob

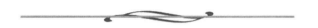

This was the week that solidified my role in this process. Heretofore, I had simply followed Charlotte's lead, tried my best to have a good attitude, and did everything I could to make her life easier. After this update, it clicked.

I knew I liked writing the updates, and the distribution list had grown significantly – to the point that I had begun to think about the size of the audience. It was daunting and unnerving. Everyone knows the idiot who sends out a mass email and totally lays an egg. The email is so bad or weird that no one even replies. I didn't want to be that guy.

I didn't know how far I should go (or could go) regarding the content, and I was very apprehensive about what I had written for this update. Did I really want to share this? Was it okay? Were my friends going to call me crazy? Were they going to slam me behind my back?

Clearly I would have never been this dramatic in my other emails about work, golf, or Texas Longhorn football.

I didn't share the content with anyone before I sent it out, but I did solicit an opinion or two regarding my hesitancy. The response was unanimously supportive. "You have done fine up to this point. Don't think about it anymore and just click send." So I did.

Within 30 minutes of the email leaving my computer, my inbox completely blew up with replies. The number of replies was very humbling and borderline embarrassing. Running around trying to be helpful on an ad hoc basis is fine and completely necessary, but finally I had a real, defined role, and it felt good to have a task. I had no idea what the weeks ahead had in store or what I would write about, but I knew I was to share the experience and I was happy to do so.

Two words: Thank You. They changed everything about my approach to the updates, and frankly, they improved my overall attitude toward life and our situation. The order of events that occurred this week was uncanny. Charlotte, my friends, and the community had no idea how intertwined they were through the words "Thank you." I was the only link to them all. Why did I feel compelled to ask my friend why he always said "Thank you" and never "Thanks"? Why did I ask him this (unbeknownst to Charlotte) prior to her thanking me before bed that night? Why did I experiment with "Thank You" all week? Why did I step out of my comfort zone and write about this in the email update? Read into it what you want to, but I think there was something larger taking place. I was led down this path with zero resistance or confrontation. The wheels were in motion to help others, to help my family, to help Charlotte heal, to give me an avenue for self-therapy, to write this book – and I had no idea. As far as I knew, all I did was write an email update that exposed some inner thoughts.

It's not chemo. It's therapy.

CHAPTER 7
I'LL HAVE A SHOT OF CONFIDENCE, A GLASS OF CHAMPAGNE AND A HAIRCUT

From: Rob Huthnance
Date: January 27, 2012 11:44:59 AM CST
To: Rob Huthnance
Subject: 1/27/12 Charlotte Update

Dear Team Charlotte,

Yesterday was Charlotte's first follow-up doctor's appointment since starting chemotherapy. He said her progress was on track and her blood counts were "perfect." Her red and white blood cells as well as her platelets were at levels equal to those of a person not currently undergoing chemotherapy. By the way, her doctor never says "chemo." When he shortens the word chemotherapy, he goes the other way and says "therapy." Her therapy yesterday was one of the long sessions, and through this morning she has had no significant issues.

I was asked yesterday by a few people, "If the blood counts are so strong, are we sure the chemo is working?" Yes, the therapy is working. We are confident of this because last Saturday she started losing her hair.

There are several homeopathic "cures" for hair loss during chemotherapy, and people love to talk about ways to keep your hair. We asked several doctors on our team about such methods. The response from them was always the same, "The drugs are designed for you to lose your hair. If you don't lose it, we will be very concerned about the effectiveness of the drugs." We decided not to pursue any remedies, and Charlotte simply embraced the idea of being bald. They told us that hair loss typically starts between days 16 and 20 after the first day of therapy.

Thompson had a basketball game Saturday afternoon. While Charlotte was getting ready for the game, she ran her fingers through her hair and ended up with several strands in her fingers. Saturday was day 16. On the way home from the game, she ran her fingers through her hair and roughly three times as many strands ended up in her fingers versus a few hours earlier. Right then she announced, "I am shaving it off today."

When we got home, I sat the children down without Charlotte in the room. We talked again about how people going through chemotherapy lose their hair. They understood. I then said, "Today is the day your mother is going to lose her hair. Would you all like to watch as we shave it off?" There was instant excitement in the room, and they couldn't wait to be part of this highly memorable event.

A few friends stopped by about this time so we decided to throw a mini-party. We popped the cork on a bottle of champagne, raised a glass to Charlotte's hair, and then we went to the back porch for the hair-cutting ceremony. We borrowed a pair of clippers, and I did the honors. First she got a number 4 cut all over, then she went "high and tight" with a number 1 on the sides and number 2 on top, and then we used just the clippers until she looked like a true Marine. As strange as it was, there were lots of laughs, high fives, and comments like, "It genuinely looks pretty good."

After this week, I am thoroughly convinced that someone with true confidence can accomplish anything. You may be dealt a difficult hand, but if you are confident on how to play the hand, you can win it.

Charlotte has had the confidence to keep on keepin' on. Being bald is now normal, and she has the confidence to accept that. We went to dinner Saturday night. She wore a hat into the restaurant, but then she had the confidence to remove it as she ate her meal. Without any hair she has had some difficulty regulating her head's temperature. She wears a hat or scarf when she gets a chill, and she takes it off when she gets hot. All with the confidence of "Hey, this is who I am. I'm very comfortable with it so everyone else should be, too."

It's fascinating how confidence makes things easier. She never frets or tries to hide the truth of the situation. I'm convinced it's this confidence, her knowing that she is being cured, that is keeping her from experiencing the typical side effects of chemotherapy.

The people from church have been very kind. The women's group this week delivered a "Basket of Sunshine." This basket contained multiple individually wrapped gifts. The gifts were to be opened whenever a little bit of sunshine was needed, and the gifts were simply items that could only put a smile on your face. This same group also constructed and placed an enormous wooden smiley face in our front yard.

This week one of the priests sent Charlotte a note. The note included a prayer from the Old Testament. When Moses' sister became sick, Moses succinctly prayed, "Please, God, please heal her."

With confidence, we are following Moses' lead and asking, "Please, God, please heal her."

Talk to you next week.

Rob

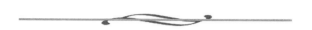

I didn't want her to shave her head. I really didn't. I never told her that, but I didn't see the harm in waiting a little longer. I'm glad, though, that I simply followed her lead. The memory of shaving her head on the porch with the children, and our friends enjoying champagne, is one that I wouldn't trade. I can't hyperbolize the level of laughter. There were no tears.

The responses I received regarding Moses' prayer were great and were all over the board. It's so simple and so easy to get your hands around. If Moses was comfortable with a five-word prayer, surely we all could be as well. That said, my favorite response was a one-word email that read: Amen.

From the time I sent the first email before her surgery, I did my best to respond to every reply I received. It often took me a couple of days, but my logic was that if someone was going to spend the time to write us a nice note, then they deserved to hear back from us.

An old friend sent the following email after reading this week's update:

> *This is strong as horseradish, buddy. I have read it about five times and I tear up each time. I have no*

doubt that Charlotte has more strength in her big toe than I do in my whole body. Peace.

I loved the "horseradish" comment. Anyone who has ever put an eighth-ounce too much on an oyster knows how strong horseradish can be. It can bring a large human to his knees. Because this was a friend I'd known since the mid '80s, I felt like I could open up a little with my response:

That's funny. She's pretty damn strong. I know it's strange, but I'm really enjoying writing these things. I get to say whatever I want and no one gets to judge me. It's a cool feeling. Obviously I wish I had a different topic to write about or could scratch the itch in another way, but these little update essays are keeping me sane and are allowing me to go places I never would have gone under different circumstances.

I hope everyone, at some point, gets to understand the feeling of being able to say whatever he or she wants without being judged. I'm not talking about First Amendment challenging stuff or anything demeaning or hurtful – just free-flow – let it out in exactly the way your brain works … and Charlotte's cancer gave me that opportunity.

Confidence is such an interesting characteristic, quality, trait, attribute, or belief. I can't pinpoint exactly what confidence is, but I know it lies somewhere amongst these five words. There is a Goldilocks and the Three

Bears aspect to it. Too much confidence is often troublesome, too little is often useless, and the right amount is just right. When you are confident about a subject or situation, nothing is troubling and there is no anxiety. On the bookends of confidence are the words timid and cocky, neither of which is enviable.

From this point forward we always tried to refer to her chemotherapy treatments as therapy – not chemo. It just sounds better. The word chemo really started to get under our skin, mine especially. It sounds sick, ill, and poisonous, while therapy sounds like anything but those words. Webster's defines therapy as "treatment to cure."

CHAPTER 8
WHY ARE WE NUMB TO SMALL VICTORIES?

From: Rob Huthnance
Date: February 3, 2012 11:55:00 AM CST
To: Rob Huthnance
Subject: 2/3/12 Charlotte Update

Dear Team Charlotte,

On Monday I had a long conversation with an old friend. He lives out of state now, and as so often is the case, we have drifted apart over the years. However, if anyone tapped the line and listened in on our conversation, they would never know how much time there had been between real conversations. Our visit was great, and I'm convinced there are many more phone calls to share in the immediate future. We talked a lot about life, and he shared how he much enjoyed the present and didn't want to live in the past. However, he mentioned that he longed for the opportunity to relive a few choice moments to better celebrate special times as they were occurring.

There is a blood test called CA 125. This test detects a protein that is found in greater concentration in ovarian cancer cells than in other cells of the body. The typical, healthy female has a level of 35 or below, and levels above 35 can give reason for concern. The doctors gave Charlotte this blood test prior to her surgery. At that time, knowing ovarian cancer was a likely diagnosis, we were hoping for a level of approximately 85. Her number came back quite high at 544.

Needless to say, the number 544 has been embedded in our minds for weeks. When we met with the doctor last week, he ran several tests, including a new CA 125. He said we wanted the results to come in no higher than 425, meaning a drop of approximately 20 percent. Given the success of the surgery and the several rounds of therapy, we found this reasonable and hoped and prayed for a good level. We anxiously awaited the results of the test, and we expected them to come back on Monday.

I spoke to Charlotte at 4 p.m. on Monday and inquired about the results. She said that she had not heard from the doctor, and we surmised that the office got busy. It was late in the day, and so we anticipated we would hear in the morning. My phone rang about a half hour later. It was Charlotte, and she said she had just gotten off the phone with the nurse.

I said, "And???" Through tears of joy, she said her number was 44.

That's a 91 percent decline! We would have been thrilled with a 25 percent decline. This is wonderful news. The plan is working.

A celebration like my friend had talked about was certainly in order.

That night when I got home, after giving her a hug, I went to the refrigerator, pulled out a bottle of champagne, popped the cork (while Georgeann covered her ears), and poured two glasses. Champagne never tasted so sweet.

My father has always been well versed at celebrating. Whether it was dinner at Luby's because I did well in Little League, a family trip to celebrate my parents' cancer remission, or a bottle of the good stuff at 3 a.m. after my announced engagement to Charlotte, he has always celebrated things in life. He has even been known to celebrate a really good Tuesday. Throughout my adult life, I have tried to follow his lead regarding celebration, but this week, celebrating became so much more important, necessary, and enjoyable.

For some strange reason celebrating – or planning a celebration – can seem arduous, and I don't know why. It should be the easiest thing in the world to do. Who doesn't like to celebrate? Why don't we do it more often? Why are we numb to small victories?

In our house, there will be no more letting victories, on any level, slip by without a focused celebration. Charlotte and I are determined to celebrate more going forward in life. It's fun to celebrate. Real fun.

Five therapy rounds are in the books. Cheers!

Talk to you next week.

Rob

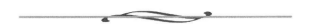

For weeks we had been so hung up on the fact that her number was 544 before surgery. That number was the only thing that we could really grasp. It was tangible. I can tell you exactly how much more 544 is than 85 or 35. Whether it's in ounces, pounds, number of sticks or cars in the parking lot, the number was real. The cancer wasn't. We never saw the scan, and we never saw the tumor. We could see the number. It's like a golf score. A high number is bad, and a low number is good. Got it.

There is no way to describe that phone call. We were so excited for what we believed was incredible news. How could we not celebrate?

My awareness of uncanny happenings is really starting to percolate. Why did I have the conversation about celebrating little events and then shortly thereafter find myself in a place where a celebration was warranted? I felt so fortunate to be able to recognize this connection, and I couldn't wait to type it out for the week's update.

I also began feeling something else about sending these updates. Pressure is not the right word for it, but given the comments from friends, and thanks to the power of the forward button, even from complete strangers, these updates were garnering some attention. I was responsible for them. I knew I couldn't knock people's socks off (or as my father-in-law says – blow their skirt up) every week, but I didn't want to let anyone down either. I became acutely aware of every conversation because I never knew when a one-liner would make me say "Hmmm … "

We have a friend who has accomplished many things in her life, including authoring a few books. "On the side" she writes a blog on the website for Runner's World magazine. After reading this week's update she sent the following email:

I love the way you write, Rob.

"Why are we numb to small victories?"

This sentence rests heavy on me and I'm going to do something about it. I love being on Team Charlotte. Thank you for the honor.

Hug your beautiful brave wife for me. Tell her I will raise a glass in her honor tonight.

What a compliment. I really appreciated her accolades as they provided adrenaline to keep moving forward with the updates. What came next, though, was a complete surprise. Her line of "This sentence rests heavy on me and I'm going to do something about it" meant the "Why are we numb to small victories?" question was going to be the topic of her blog post the following week.

When I read her blog post, I couldn't believe what I was reading. First of all, it was very humbling to read how the small victories comment struck a chord with her, and it was special to see how she transformed the thought even further. Next, I was so grateful that she associated the comment with Charlotte's fight with ovarian cancer. We are consistently focused on raising awareness for this disease, and this was a great way to do that. And finally, many of her followers posted replies saying how great Team Charlotte must be and that they would be praying for her friend named Charlotte. Come on with it. More prayers never hurt anyone.

For the record, regarding the old friend who lives out of state, he and I are totally back on track. We visit regularly, and Charlotte and I even got to have lunch with him when he was in town for a brief stay. Amazing the good that cancer can do sometimes. Keep your eyes open so you can recognize the small victories – look for them – and don't allow yourself to be numb to them. They are fun to celebrate.

CHAPTER 9
ATTITUDE IS EVERYTHING

From: Rob Huthnance
Date: February 10, 2012 12:37:05 PM CST
To: Rob Huthnance
Subject: 2/10/12 Charlotte Update

Dear Team Charlotte,

My grandfather was a typical product of the Depression and a contributing member of The Greatest Generation. He had an incredible attitude that never wavered. Ever. When teaching us about having a positive attitude, he used to say, "I like being around people, and people like being around others with a good attitude."

Yesterday an old friend flew in from Houston for the day to be with Charlotte during her therapy treatment, and I had the pleasure of picking her up at the airport and getting to visit with her first. I dropped her off at the house where she and Charlotte instantly got lost in a couple hours of conversation. I met them for lunch, and then they made the trip up the Tollway to the doctor's office.

After her therapy, we met for a drink to celebrate. Six treatments are behind us, and Charlotte is one-third through this chapter. Thank Heaven the calendar is flying by and working in our favor.

At the end of the day, I took our friend back to the airport. During the drive, the topic of conversation was how amazing Charlotte's attitude is and how powerful and infectious a good attitude is. We concluded that an upbeat attitude and positive thinking had to be key ingredients to healing.

It's not chemo. It's therapy.

Before the first round of therapy, my mother's friend constructed a "chain" made with links of construction paper. There are eighteen links in the chain. Each link represents one round of therapy. Every Wednesday night we gather as a family and break a link of the chain and place the broken link in a glass vase. It's very visual for all of us, especially the children, to see how things are progressing. Written separately on a corresponding card is a Bible verse or encouraging statement.

I had a business dinner Wednesday night and missed this week's ceremony. I should have asked how it went when I got home after the dinner, but honestly, I didn't think to ask.

Last night I was pondering what to say in this week's update. Reflecting upon the attitude conversation I'd had earlier during the car ride to the airport, I was zeroing in on that subject. Around 8:30 last night, Charlotte walked up to me, unprompted, and handed me the quote from Wednesday's link. I read the quote. It was from Charles Swindoll, and five words into it I had one of those "Are you kidding me?" moments. I don't think the attitude affirmation was happenstance.

"The longer I live, the more I realize the impact of attitude on life. Attitude, to me, is more important than facts. It is more important than the past, than education, than money, than circumstances, than failures, than successes, than what other people think or say or do. It is more important than appearance, giftedness or skill. It will make or break a company … a church … a home. The remarkable thing is we have a choice every day regarding the attitude we will embrace for that day. We cannot change our past … we cannot change the fact that people will act in a certain way. We cannot change the inevitable. The only thing we can do is play on the one string we have, and that is our attitude … I am convinced that life is 10 percent what happens to me and 90 percent how I react to it. And so it is with you … we are in charge of our attitudes."

Another friend, whose profession depends on attitude more than any other profession I know, has convinced me over the last several weeks that "Attitude is everything." I truly believe that, and by witnessing Charlotte's attitude, I recognize that it's possible, and always a choice, to have a positive attitude about anything.

Charlotte's fitness trainer, who is an awesome member of Team Charlotte, commented to me this week how great it was to see her in the gym on Tuesday. He also said he has never seen someone genuinely smile while they were doing lunges. It's an attitude. My friends who do CrossFit tell me that all the time, but I have a hard time believing them. I find my attitude is perfectly fine with a few minutes of weights and a stroll on the treadmill. Godspeed to the CrossFit guys.

Charlotte loves arts and crafts. This week she made laminated smiley faces with "Attitude is Everything" written on the back. She plans to hand them out, so be on the lookout. But be aware, if you get one, it may be because your attitude is not up to her liking. Be prepared for an attitude adjustment. She's pretty good at helping people make the adjustment – just ask our children.

And for one more smile, this week a friend persuaded George Strait, arguably the second love of Charlotte's life, to send an autographed cowboy hat, CD box set, and photo. The message on the photo was "To Charlotte, Hang in there! You are in my prayers! Love, George Strait."

Talk to you next week.

Rob

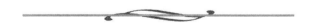

Commenting on this update is somewhat challenging for me. I do my best to put forth a good attitude to the public, but behind closed doors I often struggle with my attitude. I know being positive is the right thing to do, and I always feel better when I am upbeat. However, many events often seem out of my control, and that really stresses my attitude. Certain deals, work relationships, friendships, my golf game, sleepless nights, corked wine, new recipes that have no flavor, Charlotte's health, and my health – all can be challenging. Things seem so clear to me on how they should function; yet many times they take on a life of their own. When they do, stress kicks in and my attitude goes south.

I think in Charlotte's case a good attitude was the only choice. In her mind a bad attitude keeps you sick, and a good attitude makes you well. With traditional forces and worries that can drive attitude, the outcome of the event is rarely catastrophic, but with cancer, the worst of outcomes is possible. She focused so much of her efforts on being and remaining positive. She innately knew that if she had a smile on her face, how could anyone around her frown?

I know a lot of the attitude discussion gives the appearance that our lives were rosy during this time. Don't misconstrue the positive attitude for an easy time with cancer and therapy. It's a test, a hard test, every single day. It's a test I hope no one has to take. We had a lot of hard times, but we did our best to keep the attitude lapses and scary thoughts behind closed doors. The positive attitude we all tried to display to the community allowed the community to approach us differently. The attitude took away the "I'm so sorry" conversation and replaced it with "I'm so happy you are doing well." We fed off their support, and the circle continued.

The responses to the quote from Charles Swindoll were spot on, ranging from "That is my new screensaver" to "I have printed that out and will be taping it on the doors of my children's rooms." Attitude is everything.

This week my younger and only brother called me. Because he and his wife and their three children live in Houston, almost 250 miles away, they had some feelings of helplessness. They had been wracking their brains for weeks on ways they could provide some genuine assistance. Given the distance between Dallas and Houston, so many of the everyday things we would find helpful were just not feasible. Consequently, they went for one big thing versus multiple, smaller, practical, everyday assistance things. Their offer was unparalleled.

Once all of the therapy treatments were finished, they wanted to treat Charlotte and me to a celebration trip to the beach. It was music to our ears. We were so excited about this and loved the thought of putting sand between our toes. The trip itself was magnificent, but just having the trip on the calendar did more for us throughout her therapy than just about anything else.

Having events in the future that you can look forward to and daydream about are imperative. Being able to focus on and anticipate good things that were days, weeks or months in the future was a crucial part of maintaining general sanity and the good attitude that my grandfather and Mr. Swindoll proclaimed was so important. It's a little easier to tolerate some pain and down days when you know there is something fantastic right around the corner. This trip served as that something fantastic many, many times.

CHAPTER 10
WHAT IS CHARLITUDE?

From: Rob Huthnance
Date: February 17, 2012 11:39:36 AM CST
To: Rob Huthnance
Subject: 2/17/12 Charlotte Update

Dear Team Charlotte,

Because of this darn disease, we are now privy to countless cancer stories. While people enjoy discussing the successful ones, we are acutely aware that there are some horrific stories about cancer's capabilities. We are very close to one young boy's struggle that just flat out isn't fair. And because we are aware of others' adverse circumstances, there is a level of awkwardness in discussing how well Charlotte is doing. But our story is our story, we are so proud of her vigor, and we recognize how extremely fortunate we are.

On several occasions since Charlotte's diagnosis, I have had similar conversations with people, and specifically, I had it three times this week. Charlotte and I had the conversation with another couple after Sunday supper at their house, I had it again on Monday with an old college friend, and the topic came up over coffee on Wednesday. Each time the conversation seemed well received by both parties, so I would like to share it in this week's update.

Typically, it starts with the other party saying something to the effect of "I just can't believe how well Charlotte is doing and how well you all are handling the situation." It's a wonderful and always welcomed statement.

It's not chemo. It's therapy.

For weeks, I didn't know what else to say to the compliment other than "Thank you. She is doing really well." However, this week I found a way to expand my response with the hope of sharing further insight into our situation.

I followed up "She is doing really well" with this anecdote:

When you first realize cancer has entered your world, your house, your family, your wife, it feels like Mickey Mantle hit you in the knees with a baseball bat. Then at some point a few hours or days down the road, you realize you can handle the situation in one of two ways. You can crawl in a hole and live, breathe, and eat nothing but cancer, or you can accept the new normal, execute the plan, and keep on living.

Fortunately for us, from minute one, our community of friends gave us only one choice — keep on living. An old friend who is a physician told me early on this would happen, but he admits now that no one could have predicted the level of support we have received. We were instantly propped up by literally hundreds of people. Thankfully, all our friends were so proactive that we never had a chance to contemplate retreating into our own little world. Every time we think about those who are insisting upon our success, we acknowledge how it is the most humbling thing we have ever experienced.

Then after a few more days of living, you realize that doing everyday things feels really good. Things like working, running errands, talking on the phone, cocktailing with friends, laughing, texting a good zinger, cooking, hitting golf balls, sharing a beer, helping with homework, and writing these updates.

It's amazing how when you keep on living, cancer becomes diminished. It is absolutely a part of our lives, but it is such a smaller part of life today than it was sixty days ago. Thank goodness — because cancer sucks, and man, does it feel good to keep on living. It's so much easier. I promise.

This week Charlotte had a doctor's appointment before her therapy session. As we were driving to the doctor's office, I thought to myself how bizarrely comfortable that drive has become, how comfortable we have become with the waiting room and office environment, how comfortable we are with the staff. I had to ask myself, "Is that comfort God's grace?" I struggle with that, but I think it is. I think grace is what allows us to shift prayers from please to thank you.

The doctor visit went well. He is pleased with Charlotte's progress, and he expects her tumor markers to continue to normalize. Her white blood counts were a little low, but he was very comforting as he described how this happens to 100 percent of patients going through chemotherapy. As a result, this weekend I get to pretend I'm a medical professional and administer a couple of shots to boost her system. I hope our house doesn't turn into a M*A*S*H episode.

Early this morning when I walked outside, on the front porch was a large poster. Written across the top was "What is Charlitude?" Twenty women, some of whom I have never met, had written one-liners about Charlotte and her attitude. All were great, but one in particular made me say wow — "She has the 'I want to sit next to her, and I'll have what she's having' effect." With things like this happening regularly, how do you *not* keep on living?

There are seven rounds behind us, and this is how we are handling the situation. We made the choice a while back, and now no one is letting us change our minds. We are excited to keep on living, smiling, and laughing. Thank you for the help.

Talk to you next week.

Rob

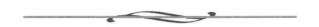

Can you believe someone came up with the word "Charlitude?" I mean come on. Really? How cool is that? We now use it as part of our daily vernacular, and I'm blown away every time I hear the word.

It never ceases to amaze us how some people handle themselves and the stories they tell. We have learned to laugh at them behind their backs. It's kinda fun. Everyone knows someone with cancer, and folks love to tell you other people's drama and sorrows. It's fascinating how many people actually tell you about some friend of theirs (whom Charlotte and I have never heard of) who was diagnosed with cancer and died. And friends think they are being helpful by doing this? Honestly. After experiencing this several times, we finally just had to start laughing. We got a kick out making fun of the storyteller later on when we were alone.

This is actually common in pregnancy, too – people often tell horror stories of tragic pregnancy problems to a pregnant woman. Probably these people are well-meaning, or perhaps they're just unconscious and unaware of the effect it can have on the listener. To anyone who has ever thought about telling a cancer patient about someone they know who also has cancer or who died of cancer, please keep your words to yourself and simply talk about the weather.

On the flip side of this, we felt guilty on several occasions for Charlotte's successful fight. When you are down to your final chips at the blackjack table in Las Vegas, the last thing you want to see is the guy on the other end of the table trying to high-five the dealer because he just won a big hand. We have met many courageous people over the last few months whose bodies had not responded to therapy in the same way Charlotte's has, or people whose cancer continues to return. That said, the truth is our story, and we certainly aren't ashamed of the truth.

I also wanted to give people a little more info beyond "she is doing fine." I figured if they asked, then I should tell them. So I started expanding a little. The additional info was well received, and the normalcy of being worried and then getting better seemed to provide some comfort to others.

I really struggled with talking about God's grace in this update; however, I felt very compelled to tell what I believed to be taking place. I have never felt as though it was my job to preach to people. There are many well-educated scholars out there better qualified than I am to do that. I'm not going to hide what I believe, and I'm happy to talk about my beliefs if asked. I didn't want to use this platform to cram religion down people's throats, but if our story made someone out there think about God, then that had to be a good thing. Wherever the reader's thoughts went from there would then be up to the reader. Our family simply wants to lead by example, as challenging and sometimes hypocritical as that may be.

It felt really good to do normal things. Just keep living. Once we got into a routine, doing ordinary things was a lot of fun. We also became keenly aware of how much fun little things could be. I love to smoke ribs, chicken, salmon, brisket, and sausage. I had no idea how much pleasure I could find in hanging out in the back yard next to the smoker with a beer or two. Charlotte swears that I actually have conversations with my smoker. She claims that when she looks through the back windows she can see me talking to it. I'm calling BS on that, but I do love my smoker. I love doing something that requires some attention and effort, yet is easy and brainless. Thank you to the friends who would stop by for a few laughs and a beer or two just because they could smell the smoke in the air.

I suspect it is similar in all parts of the country, but guys in Texas, at least it's true with all of my friends, don't feel liked unless they are being made fun of. That may sound strange, but people here don't make fun of those they don't like. It would be rude to do that. So in our circle, good-natured ribbing is welcomed and fun. Since this type of good, clean fun is all that I know, it was strange and surreal for us (me) to receive a true outpouring of love from our friends. Genuine friends are genuinely good.

CHAPTER 11
IT'S OKAY IF YOU CAN'T BREATHE

From: Rob Huthnance
Date: February 24, 2012 11:16:57 AM CST
To: Rob Huthnance
Subject: 2/24/12 Charlotte Update

Dear Team Charlotte,

I was mildly nervous going into last weekend because I was committed and scheduled to give my first injection to a human. I have given many shots to cows at the ranch, and I received allergy shots a couple times a week as a kid. I thought I knew exactly what to do. I did all of the pregame stuff perfectly – drew the medicine into the syringe, flicked all the air bubbles out, and sterilized her skin with alcohol. However, there were a few inches of fluid in the shot, and it takes several seconds to inject that much medicine. Therefore, my fears of creating a M*A*S*H episode came true. Hawkeye and Hot Lips would have been proud.

There was nothing funny about the situation, but the moment I opened the sterile packaging, I started laughing. Then once I actually pierced her skin and began pushing the plunger, Charlotte said "Ouch!" which only made me laugh harder, which made the needle wiggle around, which made her scream "Ouch!" which made me laugh harder ... and then it was déjà vu all over again twenty-four hours later as she had to have a second shot. Geez.

It truly wasn't funny, but I got a big belly laugh out of it. Sorry, Sweetheart, I'll do better next time. Luckily we have a couple of weeks for me to get my game face back.

It's not chemo. It's therapy.

At the doctor's visit last week, they performed another CA 125 test. We got the results back Tuesday morning, and the number had fallen again — from 44 three weeks ago to 29. In doctor speak, it is encouraging that her tumor marker continues to normalize. In Huthnance speak, Hell Yes!

With a level of 29 it is very clear that the doctor in fact removed the existing tumors, and the therapy is working. By definition, microscopic cancer cells remain present in the body after surgery; that is why she had to start her therapy so quickly. Statistical success rates increase dramatically if the patient can absorb the poisonous drugs as soon as possible, and 100 percent of Charlotte's follow-up tests have proven this theory correct. When coupling "Charlitude" with the effectiveness of her treatment, I almost feel sorry for her cancer cells ... but not really.

On Sunday, we attended a fundraising event for the Ovarian Cancer Research Fund. This organization specializes in the promotion of early detection of ovarian cancer. So many women who contract this disease show no symptoms and are not diagnosed until the disease has progressed significantly. The group also is determined to understand what causes ovarian cancer.

The fundraiser was a first-time event for Dallas. A few other cities have had similar events, and we benefited from their playbook. The organizers had hoped to raise $50,000 and the final tally was $285,130.

The fundraiser, named Ovarian Cycle, was a six-hour indoor cycling event, with the "cycling" on stationary bikes, or spinning cycles, sometimes called spin cycles. There was no band, no bar, and therefore no expenses. How many charity events are like that? All of the money raised will simply fight cancer.

A total of 307 participants either formed teams to ride in a "relay" or tag team for six hours or (modestly or miraculously) took it on individually. Charlotte had people do both to show their support. Kudos to all, but the individual six-hour endurance test on a stationary bike was like nothing I had seen.

Marathon runners, triathletes, and outdoor cyclists all get a change of scenery as they push themselves. When you ride 100 miles in a gym without going anywhere, all you see are the four walls of the gym and other cyclists panting, drinking water, and eating power bars. But they did it. No one quit.

Our family even left for lunch only to return to the cyclists still pedaling in the same positions on the same spin cycles.

The music on the gym system was loud. There were professional trainers offering words of encouragement and pacesetting assistance. There were pictures of women with ovarian cancer on a theater screen, and there was a banner running from the ceiling to the floor with names on it. The longest name on the banner was right there in the middle of the long column — Charlotte Huthnance. It was very sobering for me.

I was taken aback as I looked over the room. Here were a few hundred people affected in some way by ovarian cancer. Approximately 21,000 women are diagnosed annually in the United States; therefore, I recognize that others have the disease, but none of our friends do. All the support in our little world has been for Charlotte. How are there so many people out there that are in exactly the same boat? They have their own little world, doctors, support systems, struggles and wins. It was difficult for me to fathom and process that so many others were equally as mad at ovarian cancer.

I started to wish I would have ridden the six hours, but after sharing a beer and some Mexican food with our friend who rode the full six, I'm glad he did it for me. Thank you. That was a real challenge.

Eight rounds are behind us. We are six days away from the halfway point, and that sounds like a good reason to celebrate this weekend.

Talk to you next week.

Rob

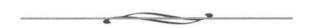

I wish someone had videoed the booster shot escapade. It really was funny. It hurt Charlotte, but she can laugh at it now. Had we videoed the scene, it would have gone viral on YouTube. It felt like we were laughing in church. Meaning you could not stop because you knew the more you laughed the more trouble you were going to be in and the harder you tried to stop, the harder you kept laughing. The plunger on the syringe was several inches long, and it takes a while to inject that much medicine. And then to do it while you are laughing hysterically, my hands just couldn't be held steady enough for it not to hurt.

The CA 125 test became a big event in our lives. It had proven to be such a barometer for her cancer, and the feeling of elation kept coming as her numbers trended lower. To start out at 544, when 35 is normal, and then to come in at 29, was beyond relief. It was such confirmation for us. The numbers don't work like that for everyone, but we were so thankful that the test worked for Charlotte.

The Ovarian Cycle event was incredible. First, what a great way to raise money, and they exceeded their goal by so much. It was a very powerful moment for me when reality hit as I read her name on the banner. I tried to be the tough guy and hang in there. There were so many people at the event trying their best for ovarian cancer funding that I was determined not to cave in to the weight of the realization.

However, I couldn't do it. The room was spinning, my breath was laboring, and I felt a major breakdown coming on. I hadn't had one in a long time, and I guess I was due. I had no idea what to do or how I was going to mask what was happening inside of me. I felt like everyone in the room was staring at me, even though I knew they weren't. I looked around and saw my youngest daughter. I immediately grabbed Georgeann, swooped her up into my arms, and we went out for a quick walk so I could catch my breath. The moment totally overwhelmed me, and I needed a break. We returned several minutes later recommitted to being strong and encouraging.

There was a guest spin cycle at the front of the room. Charlotte rode it for a few minutes and the crowd cheered like crazy. The event made the community newspaper and our family's picture and Charlotte's story were front and center. The kids loved seeing their picture in the paper.

When he heard about this event, Charlotte's little brother wanted to participate. He is in good shape, so an event like this suited him well. However, what really touched Charlotte was that several of her brother's friends wanted to participate as well. She had been a "big sister" to so many of his friends over the years, and this was a very nice way for them to show their gratitude.

Our friend who rode the full six hours had approached us weeks earlier and said he wanted to do something for Charlotte, and this was something he could do. He admitted also that he was looking forward to losing a little weight, which would inevitably occur given the amount of training required to ride 100 miles. He has been successful raising money for charities in the past, and he believed he could help this cause as well. He raised several thousand dollars, spread awareness, and enlisted support from people who had been out of our lives for a long time. When I read the contributors list, I had several moments when I thought, "I can't believe they contributed in Charlotte's honor." Before cancer entered our lives, I'm not sure I would have supported a cause in their honor had the situation been reversed. I'm not sure what that says about me, but I know what it says about them.

CHAPTER 12
THE TRUTH SHALL SET YOU FREE

From: Rob Huthnance
Date: March 2, 2012 10:02:28 AM CST
To: Rob Huthnance
Subject: 3/2/12 Charlotte Update

Dear Team Charlotte,

I went to second semester summer school before my freshman year at the University of Texas. My second day on campus I walked past the Tower, the main building at the center of campus. I looked up and read the statement chiseled into the façade – "Ye shall know the truth, and the truth shall set you free."

I remember being completely in awe and I stood there staring at the building, the words, the campus, the people, and I absorbed the energy. I considered that statement as an eighteen-year-old thinking I was old and mature but knowing I had my entire life in front of me. I wanted to know the truth, and I wanted to feel that feeling of freedom that the statement promised.

In the twenty-something years since, I don't know that I know the truth or have found the truth, but telling the truth about our family's situation has been an extremely freeing process for me. Being open, honest, and (I hope) informative about Charlotte's cancer has proven to be a comfortable approach. Because we haven't tried to cover up what's actually happening, we don't have to hide behind cancer. And the best thing about telling the truth is how the truth has helped our children deal with and understand Mommy's situation. They feed on Charlitude.

Numerous friends and people who were strangers before Charlotte's diagnosis have asked me about the updates. How do you come up with the words? Did you know you could write? Do you write fancy Valentines to Charlotte?

Hallmark always writes my cards, and usually her Valentine is the funniest one I can find at the drug store in less than ninety seconds. Some cards are better than others, and Charlotte can probably name the best ones from memory.

The honest answer to the writing question is that writing comes naturally when you are just telling the truth. I have always enjoyed writing on some level. I have written mandatory term papers, investment memos for work, and the occasional (often obligatory) thank-you note. Other than that, I never really had anything to write about until now. It's strange how people get led down paths they never dreamed they would follow. I feel led down this path to communicate with everyone about Charlotte's cancer, and I'm thrilled that so many people have an interest in her well-being.

Monday morning Charlotte was sitting at a stoplight. A woman pulled up next to her and rolled down her window. Charlotte rolled her window down, thinking the woman was going to ask for directions. Instead the woman said, "I have seen smiley faces all over town, and I figured you would know what they are for, since you have several on the back of your car. Can you please tell me?" Surprised, Charlotte replied, "They are for me. I was diagnosed with ovarian cancer, and I am going to smile my way through it." The cars behind them started honking, and they drove their separate ways.

On Tuesday, my mother and two of her friends flew in from Austin for the day. They went to lunch and did a little shopping. I wasn't invited to the party. They had a wonderful time, and Charlotte certainly appreciated the effort. The trip was planned six weeks ago, and the women's original intention was to attend to

Charlotte at her bedside. At the time of the booking, no one contemplated a nice lunch and shopping. My mother later told me that the conversation on the flight home was how they came up to comfort Charlotte, and instead Charlotte was a comfort to them. They knew she was doing well. They had heard the stories and read the weekly updates, but sometimes you just have to see it to believe it. They are now believers.

Charlotte had a big day on Tuesday because that evening several of the moms from Georgeann's school hosted a manicure, pedicure, and pizza party at the nail salon. Charlotte had bright yellow polish painted on her toes and smiley faces added to both big toes. The smiley faces are almost ridiculous, but they are still very fun and put a little pep in your step every time you see one.

Yesterday, for the first time since December 8th, I took a day trip for business. I even got to fly on an airplane. The day went well, and the trip was productive. It was refreshing to be on the road. I was able to get away on a Thursday because an old friend from San Antonio came in to accompany Charlotte to her therapy session.

Thursday before Charlotte's therapy, they went for a walk and solved lots of the world's problems, then made the familiar trip to Plano. The nurse had to take a mulligan again on the IV. That's now five out of nine times which is very frustrating and painful. Otherwise the session went off without a hitch. On the way home, the girls couldn't help themselves and stopped off for a celebratory champagne toast.

Charlotte finished the front nine this week and has made the turn a couple strokes under par. She tees off on number 10 next Thursday at 11 a.m. Just need to stay focused and bring it on home.

Talk to you next week.

Rob

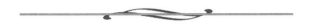

These updates started out with me sitting at my computer for a few minutes on Friday morning and typing as fast as my brain could think of words. I would write out the update, let it sit for a couple of hours, reread it a couple of times, tweak a word or two and click send. As time continued, I was asked by several people how much time I was devoting to these updates. I never felt as though I was spending that much time on them, but I understood the question. I started to time them just to see. Updates 3 through 5 averaged around twenty minutes. The brevity surprised some people, but a couple of close friends guessed the updates didn't absorb a lot of my time. They knew me well enough to know – this is just how my brain works.

A few weeks into this process I started to take my job a little more seriously. A lot of people were actually reading these things. Over the last couple of months at every social engagement, the first thing out of people's mouths was "How's Charlotte?" and the second thing was something about the updates. I felt like I had to address it directly, and the truth topic enabled me to do that. It also just happened to fit this week. The quote chiseled on the tower façade was the most direct way I could discuss what truth was and what it meant to me. Who doesn't want to be set free?

The stoplight story is one of Charlotte's favorites. Everything about it just worked. The woman made Charlotte feel good because she had noticed all the smiley faces, and because the light turned green, Charlotte didn't have to come up with an abundance of small talk.

My wife does not particularly wear polish on her fingernails, but she loves having her toes painted. I think she likes the pageantry of the pedicure more than the polish. She likes sitting in a plush, comfortable chair, listening to soothing music, not having any little people tugging at her, soaking her feet, having someone massage them, and then, just out of obligation to have a closing ceremony, getting them painted. The smiley face toenails were fun. Springtime is pleasant in Dallas, and you can see the toes of just about any girl or woman at any given moment. Flip-flops or sandals rule the scene. Having smiley faces on her toes was a unique and personal twist that gave a charge to lots of folks throughout the day.

Getting out of town on a 12-hour business trip was probably the most refreshing and energizing thing I had done. It was just for me. I love being at the 19th hole with my friends, but the topic of conversation was always the same. Out of town, no one knew that my wife was sick. When I got home late that night, I was ready to get back at it and help Charlotte annihilate cancer.

The IV thing did get to be old. You just wanted the nurses to get it right the first time. A couple of the nurses commented, or complained, about her not having a port. A port is a temporary, permanent needle that remains in your chest for the entire duration of your chemotherapy treatments. It makes it very convenient to plug back into the drip IV week to week, but when you are not at the doctor's office receiving treatment, it serves as a constant reminder that you are sick. It is always there. Charlotte chose early on to not have a port installed. She would endure the weekly needle pricks, and the misses, to not have the constant reminder.

Whenever an out-of-towner came in to accompany Charlotte to therapy, the day was simply brighter. She (we) so appreciated the effort, and it was great to see a friend that we were unable to see regularly because of geography. Moreover, when a local friend would go with her, a level of guilt often came with the trip. Carpools and children's activities had to be covered by someone else, and you just felt guilty knowing the mom in charge was only a few miles away. The level of commitment taken on by an out-of-towner made the situation feel easier. She couldn't watch the clock and stress over carpool. There was nothing she could do from a few hundred miles away. The only clock watching was at the end of the day to make sure she didn't miss the airplane home.

The champagne toasts on the way home from the doctor were fun. They made Charlotte feel alive and were the perfect punctuation mark on a successful therapy session.

CHAPTER 13
GO AHEAD AND TELL GOD WHAT YOU WANT

From: Rob Huthnance
Date: March 9, 2012 11:08:58 AM CST
To: Rob Huthnance
Subject: 3/9/12 Charlotte Update

Dear Team Charlotte,

You ever try telling God what to do? In my lifetime, I have prayed that way a handful of times. Time will tell how it works out for me, but that is exactly what a woman did for Charlotte last Sunday night.

We had gone out to eat Mexican food, and somehow Charlotte left her phone in the car – that never happens. When we finished and got the kids loaded up, Charlotte picked up her phone. It showed a voicemail from an "Unknown" caller.

Charlotte has a friend who is friends with the sister of a world-famous preacher. The preacher's sister somehow got their mother to call Charlotte. I know all of those relationships make your head spin, but it's necessary to paint the picture. Feel free to reread it, it's a little confusing. The preacher's mother obviously knows a thing or two about prayer given the beliefs, abilities, and massive following of her son.

Knowing nothing of what Charlotte is listening to on her voicemail, I pay it no mind and start backing out of the parking space and driving through the parking lot. Before I reach the street, she puts the phone to my ear and says listen to this! So I do. I hear the voice and the lady's name, and I look at Charlotte with the look of "Is this for real?" She nods yes. There was total communication without actually saying anything.

I listened to the message as I drove down the street. There were all the typical well wishes for someone with cancer. Then she says "I want to pray for you, and since you can't be on the phone right now, I want to pray on your voicemail."

With this, she starts telling God what to do. I mean telling him as is in "God, I need a miracle from you. You have said that you love everyone the same. You healed me in the past, you have healed lots of people with cancer, and now I want you to heal Charlotte." I know many spiritual people are proficient at praying this way, and their testimonies are always very positive.

The only other time I have witnessed anything on par with this was several years ago in what seems now like another lifetime. I was working for a large publicly traded company, and the CEO was in Dallas one day and stopped by my office to catch up. While sitting across my desk from me, he received a phone call from a United States Senator wanting to know about how a certain bill could affect the nation's commercial real estate market. Without hesitation, he starts telling the Senator exactly how he feels and precisely to the decimal point what the Senator should do. I sat there stunned and listened to what seemed to be way more instruction than the Senator had bargained for. When he got off the phone, the CEO looked at me and said, "Senators do better with some coaching. You have to tell them what you want."

However, this wasn't a Senator being directed on Charlotte's voicemail, this was God. But I suspect God knew what he was getting with this woman when he created her. I like the role she is playing, and I like the fact that God allows her, and probably encourages her, to speak to him like that. Welcome to Team Charlotte, Ma'am.

I know this is not surprising, but Charlotte is friends with all of the checkout people at the grocery store. With three kids, she is there several times a week. This week one of the women looked at her and asked, "Is there something I should know about? Why is that scarf on your head?" Charlotte's response was, "I was sick, but now I'm better and I have to continue taking medicine for a couple more months, just to be sure." The checkout woman said, "Well, I'll be praying for continued expectations."

I received an email this week from a friend whom I have not seen in a while. He has been keeping up with us via the updates. In the email, he said he saw George W. Bush speak at a charity event over the weekend. During the speech, Mr. Bush said the most surprising thing about his presidency was realizing the awesome power of prayer he and Laura had experienced while in office.

Yesterday I read that if you claim God's promises from Scripture, prayer is as simple as presenting a check and asking for cash. We had a pretty powerful week. Prayer was certainly the theme.

I have been officially relieved of my medical duties. A friend who is a registered nurse was kind enough to drop by on both Saturday and Sunday to give Charlotte the injections that increase her white blood cell count. Charlotte asked her to tell her when she was going to give the shot, only to hear "It's already done." I know my attempts were below average, but this made me look downright pitiful.

Charlotte's doctor's appointment went well yesterday. He walked into the room, asked how she was doing, and said her blood counts looked fine. We will get the results on yesterday's CA 125 test next week, and we are hoping for a number below twenty. As the saying goes, "if the trend is your friend," the number should be there. The doctor asked if we had any questions. We said no. Then he laughed and said he wished he could come up with something to discuss, but since Charlotte is in such good shape, there just wasn't much to say. We stood up, all smiled and walked down the hall to the infusion suite. This week was a long session, and she was able to sleep through most of it. Ten treatments are behind us.

Last night was Open House at the elementary school, and we bumped into a dear friend who has been such a blessing for us. Twelve months ahead of Charlotte, she annihilated her own cancer. She saw Charlotte across the hall and said, "Wasn't today a long one?" "Yep," was the answer. The comeback was then, "Dammit, it's not fair for you to feel as well as you do." Only winners get to talk to each other like that.

The preacher's mother who prayed for Charlotte ended her prayer with, "Lord I don't know Charlotte, but I know I need her in my life." Yes, Ma'am. We all do.

Talk to you next week.

Rob

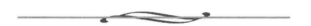

This week was very comfortable and reassuring. The phone call from the preacher's mother was pretty incredible, and really gave us a sense of the magnitude of our support platform. There were lots of people out there cheering for Charlotte, and members of Team Charlotte were even willing to recruit new members. It took some effort to pass along Charlotte's cell phone number.

Looking back, the neatest thing about the phone call was that we missed the live conversation. Charlotte is never without her phone. I have no idea how she could have forgotten it in the car. Since she didn't answer the phone and received the voicemail, we were able to listen to the message several times and even share it with others.

The power of prayer is amazing. There are times when prayers don't get answered in your requested manner or timeframe, and I wish I had a more tangible answer about why that is. Faith in knowing that God knows best is the only answer I have. It is also uncanny how often the Lord makes his presence felt when many people pray for a common cause. His presence is known in a way that says "I've got your back, keep trying your best, look to me for guidance and my plan will ultimately make you happier than you ever dreamed possible."

This week's doctor's visit was pretty funny. I can only imagine how some of those appointments go for oncologists. After witnessing the diagnosis and treatment of cancer, I know there are people who live every waking moment trying to come up with new questions for their doctor. Then every few weeks the doctor has to sit and answer all the questions the patient concocted between visits. All jobs have parts that are not necessarily enjoyable, and I suspect answering mundane and off-the-wall questions from patients is high on that list for an oncologist. Our appointment this week put a smile on the doctor's face. He looked at the blood charts said, "Okay, do you have any questions?" We said, "Nope." He got a big smile on his face and said, "Okay then." I'm sure he was thrilled to have twenty minutes put back into his day.

Throughout this process, I have loved watching Charlotte and our friend who recently beat cancer toggle back and forth. Of course, her husband and I have been privy to many conversations, and we even contributed to a couple of them. However, when I got to be a fly on the wall and just watch, it was truly special. She came over for a glass of wine the night of Charlotte's first therapy session. They sat, compared notes, and laughed while I listened in from the other room. There is just something about a bond created through strife, hardship, and determination. I have a similar bond with other "caregivers", but our bond is not as cementing as the bond of warriors and survivors.

CHAPTER 14
GOD BLESS GEORGE STRAIT

From: Rob Huthnance
Date: March 16, 2012 12:23:24 PM CDT
To: Rob Huthnance
Subject: 3/16/12 Charlotte Update

Dear Team Charlotte,

The kids were out of school this week for spring break. We spent last weekend at the ranch, and this was our first venture away from Dallas since Thanksgiving. It was wonderful to get out of town, even though it was a fairly quick trip. We really didn't do anything extraordinary or unusual, but looking back, a lot happened. We rode horses, we received positive results for Charlotte's latest CA 125 test, she had another round of therapy, and oh yeah, we had a family photo made with George Strait.

It poured down rain all day Saturday, an inch and three-quarters to be exact. With the drought everyone in Texas has experienced the last couple of years, it is socially acceptable to brag about rain. Needless to say we were thrilled to receive the rain, but we needed a rainy day activity other than sitting around the ranch house.

Some good friends of ours from San Antonio came to the rescue. They sponsor George Strait's Team Roping Classic, and they invited us to come to the event and bring the children. The event is held each year in Boerne, just northwest of San Antonio. We arrived at the arena with enough time to see the last dozen or so contestants. The winning team was as excited as anyone in the world on Saturday as they won a check for $203,000, and each received a new truck and horse trailer.

After the festivities, we got to meet George and hang out with him for a few minutes. He was very nice, and we snapped a couple of photos with him. Since each of our children has listened to his music since the day they got home from the hospital, they understood what was taking place. I'm confident this memory will be one they remember for the rest of their lives. I know Charlotte will.

This occasion presented Charlotte and me with a proud parenting moment. When we walked into the room, our son went directly to George, stuck out his hand, looked him in the eye and introduced himself. It was perfect. As we were leaving, George pulled our mutual friend aside and said, "That boy's pretty good, isn't he?" Admittedly, that's bragging. Thank you for tolerating my transgression.

For the rest of the weekend at the ranch, the weather was perfect and we simply enjoyed doing nothing. Nothing included smoking a pork butt, going on a jeep ride, riding horses in the ring, feeding the cows, roasting marshmallows, listening to a friend play guitar by the campfire, and getting some much-needed rest. All of us were perfectly content, especially Charlotte.

Charlotte called the doctor Monday morning for the results of last week's CA 125 test. We wanted a number below 20, the results had been trending that way, and the nurse told her the latest number was 18.

By now, Charlitude has been well documented. She tries hard every day to beat this disease. However, when Charlotte told me the number was 18, it was the first time that her face truly showed some sign of relief.

There was no more "I have to get through this," no more "fake it till you make it," no more "I'm not going to let anything get me down." The look of ultra determination that we have all become so accustomed to finally faded. She had the "I didn't read the chapter, and the teacher didn't call on me" look of relief — times one hundred. Deep breaths and hugs went all around.

Given the rapid descent of her tumor markers and how well she is dealing with chemotherapy, it feels as though this disease is behind us. Faith and spirit say that's correct; science says don't quit now. We clearly recognize that cancer is challenging; therefore, we are not letting up on the high dose of chemotherapy or the attitude.

Our focus for the next several weeks is somehow forcing the therapy to find any and all microscopic cancer cells that could be hiding. Again science says these hidden cells may exist, but we are confident that if there are any cancer cells left in her body, the drugs will destroy them. Her tumor marker didn't drop from 544 to 18 without confidence.

Her therapy session this week was successful. It was a one-needle event, and this week was a short session. Eleven treatments are complete.

George Strait recorded the song "Easy Come, Easy Go" twenty years ago, and the jukebox at Abel's in Austin played it regularly. I sang along to the song many, many times. Funny how I had no idea then that he was singing about the cancer in my future wife's body.

> *Goodbye, farewell, so long*
> *Vaya con Dios*
> *Good luck, wish you well, take it slow*
> *Easy come, girl, easy go*

Talk to you next week.

Rob

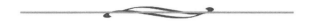

Ever since Charlotte and I first met, we traveled a lot on the weekends. Typically we went out of town a couple of times each month. Being forced to stay in Dallas was a new experience for us. On one hand it was nice to not have to load up the Suburban with all of the family's gear and spend a few hours on the highway, but at the same time we really missed escaping our routine.

The ranch is a special place for our whole family. We love spending time there, and we were so grateful for these few days.

Charlotte has had a crush on George Strait since 1982. We are fortunate enough to have a few memories of George. While we were dating we attended a concert of his in Birmingham, Alabama. We had good seats close to the stage. The stage was in the center of the large arena, and it went around and around like a Lazy Susan table in perpetual motion. When he sang "I Can't See Texas From Here," Charlotte hooked her horns as if she were cheering for a touchdown at a Texas Longhorn football game. George noticed her doing this, stopped strumming his guitar for a second, hooked his horns and pointed at her. It was pretty cool. Thanks to our mutual friends, we also have been able to sneak backstage a time or two after his concerts.

I know everyone thinks their kids are the best, and hearing stories about how great someone else's children are can be tiresome. But I just had to share that moment about Thompson. He acted like he was six feet tall instead of four foot something. I was very proud, and then to have George actually comment on it was a great slap on the back.

The good news on Charlotte's CA 125 test was very welcomed. She truly took a deep breath and felt as if all was going to be okay. This was a genuine moment, and the moment was a first. It wasn't that she was scared prior to these results, but there is no denying that we all were anxious and fearful. It's a daily struggle to not live looking over your shoulder. A positive report was encouraging affirmation and provided a quick break from the anxiety. As hard as it was, we have done our best to live day to day. We've had no idea what tomorrow would be like, so we've relished what we knew was fact for each day.

I'm not sure if the email readers kept up with me ending the update with the lyrics to "Easy Come, Easy Go" but I like that song and thought it captured the moment. I really did used to sing along with it practically nightly at Abel's, my favorite bar just west of the University of Texas campus in Austin.

It's not chemo. It's therapy.

CHAPTER 15
OUR ROUTINE IS SIMPLE: WASH, RINSE, REPEAT

From: Rob Huthnance
Date: March 23, 2012 10:40:43 AM CDT
To: Rob Huthnance
Subject: 3/23/12 Charlotte Update

Dear Team Charlotte,

I sat down at my computer to write this week's update and stared at the screen. Within ten seconds, a bird flew into my office window. This happens from time to time so I didn't pay it much attention. Then it flew into the window again and again and again — seven times total. I have no idea what was so inviting in the glass' reflection. At the very least you would think the real bird would try to dodge the other bird flying straight at it, but here it was doing the same thing over and over and over. We are at the stage in the treatment process where our lives seem similar to the actions of the bird.

Medically, we are doing the same thing over and over again each week. Going to Plano for the therapy treatments feels a little like the movie Groundhog Day — every Thursday is the same. We get in the car, drive up the Tollway, park in the same area, check in, get blood drawn, wait in the waiting room, get called back, hope for a good chair in the corner while we make the trek to the infusion suite, get situated, take the needle, approve the medicine, get sleepy from the pre-game Benadryl, swap the IV bags a few times, pack up, tell the nurses goodbye, walk out, and drive home.

Oddly, doing the same thing over and over can be comforting. Unlike the bird, we know we are doing the right thing. By all accounts the medicine is working, and Charlotte is on track for a full recovery. As she has made it through twelve treatments, we are committed to the routine six more times.

I don't know of anything else in which we are so committed to the same routine. I try to do the same thing over and over again with my golf swing, but even that gets thrown out the window from time to time — albeit mostly unintentionally. However, the result of varying my swing routine often means my next shot will require something different to help maneuver around or through an obstacle.

Everything else we encounter in life is consistently changing, and when life does become routine, we look for a change. We embrace new projects at work, new friends, new experiences, new activities for our children, new clothes, new places to travel, new wine, new recipes, new restaurants, and new stories. Who wants to hear the same joke every week for eighteen weeks? No one.

It's somewhat surreal to accept monotony, but in our case, as long as monotony ensures we will have the ability to experience wonderful, exciting new things in the not-so-distant future, we will gladly endure it. Additionally, this monotony has somehow made the calendar speed along. We live each week to get past Thursday. That's it, and when we get there, we celebrate that fact and ride out the time until the next Thursday. Wash, rinse, repeat — my buddies in Arkansas call this the shampoo effect, but they associate this process with drinking beer and not chemotherapy.

I don't want to be so bold as to say that Charlitude took a hit this week because that is not a true statement, but having a good attitude was certainly tested. In thinking through events that could be labeled monotonous yet still have great endings, I came up with a few. When a football team gains four yards every play, they score a touchdown every drive. The sun always rises in the east and sets in west, magnificently whenever you take the time to watch it. Inch by inch the caterpillar crawled onto the ark, and drip-by-drip Charlotte's cancer is being eliminated.

We know we can't go around it, over it, or under it. We have to go through it. This upcoming week, we are excited about getting to Wednesday night. Because with the comedy night scheduled in Charlotte's honor to raise money for the Mary Crowley Cancer Research Center, we will get to laugh our way to Thursday.

Talk to you next week.

Rob

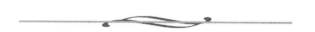

After writing this update and sending it on, the bird came back. He flew into the window a couple of times and then flew away. I don't want to read too much into a silly bird, but he did provide a calming, reassuring sense of reflection for me. His presence opened my mind to be able to see more than simply what we were living from day to day. We had been banging our heads against the wall just trying to stay on top of life. After watching him literally bang his head, I tried harder to see beyond next Thursday. I started to see what life would be like without cancer, and I understood how much more we had to endure. The end was closer than ever before, and I recognized that there was an end.

Monotony is challenging for us. As we have matured, we enjoy spending our time and money chasing new experiences. I don't need one other trinket or thing for the house, but I crave watching the sunset from a new vantage point or sharing a cocktail in a new setting with friends or feeling new and different sand between my toes. I like brainstorming for new ideas and solutions at work, and I enjoyed writing updates on different topics each week during Charlotte's treatment.

I received an email this week that did give me a reality check regarding monotony, and I appreciated the writer's spin. "Things may seem monotonous to you but not to those of us who wait expectantly for your weekly update on Charlotte's therapy. We are encouraged by knowing things are routine there and that there have been no 'surprises' thus far."

My friends from Arkansas are awesome people. We banter back and forth about pretty much everything. No topic is sacred, and anything funny is fair game. There is not much love lost between our football teams, and it's a shame we don't get to play each other more often. One of my friends from Little Rock so dislikes Texas football that when he built his house he installed a tile with a Longhorn logo upside down in his son's shower right at eye level. He is convinced that this is good parenting.

I have watched them laugh about the shampoo effect for years, and I couldn't catch my breath as I typed those words. I was all by myself and my shoulders were going up and down like pistons. I know that this kind of silly BS won't translate for a lot of people, but I promise it's funny.

With two-thirds of the treatments behind us, Charlotte and I opened up more to each other and discussed the dynamics of various friendships we have. We have been blessed with so many friends. However, when troubling times such as cancer occur, many friendships change. We noticed how some friends came out of the starting gate so fast and were ever-present in the beginning but completely faded away by the end. Others loomed in the background waiting for things to slow down before stepping in. Many, many stuck by us every single step of the way, yet some close friends, feeling very uncomfortable with our situation, pulled away entirely. There are no hard feelings, and we now understand that friends handle things differently, often in ways that are surprising. Had we tried to pinpoint the various categories friends would fall into, we would have guessed wrong many times. And not from a lack of trying – we found that relationships could not be forced. You can't let this bog you down. Be patient, don't get your feelings hurt, and allow relationships to run their course.

I did Charlotte an injustice by writing "Charlitude took a hit this week." I wanted to convey her weariness in the process. It was hard and challenging to stay on top from week to week, and this week was especially hard. Nothing new was happening and the grind was just that, a grind. I should have said things differently or not mentioned anything at all about her attitude. She received several calls from people asking what had happened this week and whether she was all right. Of course she was fine, but the added stress of having to confirm this to friends was not fair to her.

The comedy night had been in the works for weeks. One of the mom's from the children's elementary school is a professional comedian. She's hilarious. As a way to give back to the community, she organizes comedy events for charity. There is a local comedy club that helps sponsor the events, and she enlists fellow comedians willing to participate for peanuts because this is a great way for them to try out new material. The charity gets the gate, the club gets the drinks, and the comedians get feedback on what's really funny. Everybody wins.

We were so excited when she asked Charlotte in January about hosting one of these comedy events in her honor. The friend handled all the logistics. The only thing Charlotte had to do was contribute some email addresses for invitations. We had seen her act before and knew that it got pretty raunchy. We expected it would be funny, but we were a little anxious about how personal some of the jokes might be. A couple hundred tickets had been sold, and we couldn't wait for the big night.

CHAPTER 16
EVERYONE HAS PEAKS AND VALLEYS

From: Rob Huthnance
Date: March 30, 2012 2:09:50 PM CDT
To: Rob Huthnance
Subject: 3/30/12 Charlotte Update

Dear Team Charlotte,

I had a drink with an old friend this week. We had not shared a drink in quite some time, but anyone eavesdropping would never have guessed it. He's a great twenty-something-year friend. We talked about everything under the sun, but Charlotte's situation was a large part of the conversation. In the history of man, no one has enjoyed the moment more than this guy. Ask anyone. No matter the group's dynamics, he offers unequaled effervescence. It's fun to watch and be around. He gets Charlitude in a way the rest of us can't.

He talked a lot about life and the peaks and valleys we all experience, and when you recognize that things are going well, you should take a time-out and enjoy the view from the peak. Each of these elevated moments is inherently good. But in time, reality will assert itself, and you will descend to the valley; so you have to enjoy every moment from the peak while you can. That's life. It's the same for all of us.

Everyone in life has problems. Everyone experiences marital strife, money challenges, family issues, kid issues, work issues, health issues, social issues, and cars that break down. All are huge setbacks at the time, and are extremely important and frustrating to each individual. Each person's problems feel really big to them.

Charlotte and I have grown immensely in this regard. While we have had many, many issues over the years, so many of the things we thought were problems aren't even a blip on the radar screen anymore. Thank goodness, and we don't miss them.

Our current issue is cancer, but frankly, as challenging as it is, has been, and will be for a short time longer, it's only a life issue. On some level stress is stress. The feeling of stress we are experiencing feels like the same stress I've experienced countless times before her diagnosis. It took me a while to be able to admit that, but it's true. Everyone experiences sleepless nights. Everyone worries about something. That's just part of the deal we signed up for when we were born. I don't think we should feel bad about stress, but we darn sure better deal with it directly. Don't settle down in the valley. Start enjoying the view as you climb back up.

Wednesday night we thoroughly enjoyed the view along the ascent. It was comedy night, and the crowd's sides probably still hurt from laughing. Needless to say, the event in Charlotte's honor was a huge success. All the proceeds went to the Mary Crowley Cancer Research Center, the organization facilitating Charlotte's clinical trial for the cancer vaccine. Over 300 people came, and the crowd gave Charlotte and the host a standing ovation at the end of the night. All in attendance deserve a standing ovation, because enough money was raised to provide chemotherapy treatments for five people. This is how the Center is going to use the money. How cool is that? How blessed are those five people and everyone who knows them? Don't you wish you could be the one who gets to call those five people and share the good news? Way to go friends! That's how charity giving is supposed to work. Thank you.

The doctor's appointment on Thursday went well. Her blood counts are doing fine, and we will get the result of the latest CA 125 test next week. Unfortunately, she is experiencing some minor neuropathy in her hands. This is concerning because the tingling and numbing sensations can be permanent, and it will become progressively worse if not addressed now. The doctor adjusted the dosage of one of the drugs, and we hope that will do the trick.

One of Charlotte's old friends came in for comedy night and to go with her to therapy yesterday. She is such a good human. She's always helpful, loves to have fun, and knows how to celebrate. We celebrated "lucky 13" this week. Five more to go.

When you are in a valley, by definition there is a peak on the far side, and if you keep going, you can start your ascent again. When you get to the top, the view has to be better than that of the previous peak. Someone made that promise. I can't say yet what the view from the next peak will be; however, I know the ascent can be fun. Just ask one of the friends who laughed with us on Wednesday night.

Talk to you next week.

Rob

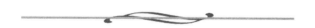

For a couple of weeks, I had been thinking about a way to incorporate the idea that stress feels like stress and you can choose to deal with it or not. It is your choice. I didn't know how to do that, and then I had a drink with my friend and he started talking about peaks and valleys.

The topics seemed to gel pretty well, so I wrote about them in this week's update.

Charlotte and I had learned on the fly that dealing directly with the major issue at hand made so many of the other outstanding issues easier to manage. It sounds easy to do, and I feel like I can multi-task pretty well, but we had not managed cumulative stress very effectively prior to cancer. Given our focus on her healing, reducing our focus on nitpicky items was easy to do, and this reduction enabled us to breathe easier than ever before.

As we have grown throughout Charlotte's time with cancer, the single most recognizable thing within our relationship is that we have a better sense of what is important. We don't raise our voices over much anymore, and we can talk openly about anything. We still aren't perfect, but living with each other is much easier.

Weeks after this update went out, I learned that it helped a friend of a friend (a person I did not know) during her substance abuse treatment. The peaks and valleys discussion resonated with her. I was blown away by that. I can comprehend how someone who struggles with substance abuse has peaks and valleys, but that never crossed my mind as I wrote the update.

Hearing about the ways these updates have helped people continuously inspires both Charlotte and me. We hoped all along that her body's ability to beat cancer would encourage others, but we had no clue that these updates would also serve as inspiration. We are glad that marrying her health with the updates might make life's roads a little less bumpy for folks who witness our story.

The comedy night was hysterical. The invite list was not necessarily exclusive, because the night was about raising money to fight cancer, but invitations were sent to people who love to laugh. We wanted a raucous crowd, knowing the crowd would make the event, no matter how funny the comedians were. Luckily, the comedians did their part and put on great performances. The crowd's laughter did the rest. Walking out, everyone was exhausted, in a good way, from laughing and cheering and giving Charlotte a standing ovation – just because they cared about her. We also love how the money was spent. Really, how fun those phone calls must have been – both making them and receiving them – with the message about free treatment.

Charlotte's old friend from college who came to visit is such a blessing to us, and she loves to laugh. She and Charlotte can finish each other's sentences, and they are so good for each other. She is the same college friend who came into town for Charlotte's surgery. Keep in mind the surgery was December 20, she has four children, and that day was her birthday. During that visit, the greatest gift she gave me was packing Charlotte's bag for the hospital. If she hadn't been here, I would have had to help Charlotte by answering a list of questions, and no matter the answers, they would have been wrong. But with me out of the picture, each answer the two women came up with was perfectly correct.

CHAPTER 17
CANCER CAN MAKE YOU BETTER

From: Rob Huthnance
Date: April 6, 2012 9:54:34 AM CDT
To: Rob Huthnance
Subject: 4/6/12 Charlotte Update

Dear Team Charlotte,

Over the last few months, many people have assured me that God always redeems what he allows. I like thinking of challenging earthly events as allowances versus mandates. I have never subscribed to the notion that God made Charlotte sick, but clearly he allowed cancer to form in her body.

My father has told me a few times over the years that the most difficult thing he encountered as a parent was choosing what to ignore. Undoubtedly, God knows what to ignore, and he chose to ignore cancer for us.

I know this sounds strange, but we are happier today with cancer in our lives than we were six months ago when we couldn't even contemplate such a challenge. We are nicer to each other, our children seem more inspired, we are more optimistic about the future, we laugh harder, cocktails taste better, we express emotions, and we celebrate exponentially more often.

For some reason, this week brought out the best in several people. We have two friends who don't know each other. They are in vastly different industries, yet this week both of them happen to be experiencing pinnacles in their careers. Yesterday, each one of them, individually, put these monumental professional events on the back burner because "Charlotte's effort yesterday was more important." It was very humbling for us because we know how important each event is to the rest of the world.

A few people dropped gifts by the house this week. The gifts were great. None was expensive, but the givers put an incredible amount of thought and effort into them. Charlotte was graciously moved in different ways by each one. Inexpensive gifts that require genuine inspiration are more fun to receive. I love saying, "How did they come up with that?"

Yesterday she went to therapy with a friend, who wrote her a real poem, and not some silly poem used by sorority sisters during rush. This one was the real deal and very fun to read. Then after therapy they went to a "party" on the patio at the Ritz, where they celebrated with champagne. It was a glorious day in Dallas, which made celebrating outside that much more fun.

Charlotte has befriended a new nurse in the infusion suite, and she is now two for two on getting the needle placed with one try. We are very grateful for her ability. Charlotte's numbers continue to be outstanding. Her CA 125 test came back on Monday. The number was 13.

It's a bizarre revelation to be grateful for cancer; however, that's where we find ourselves. Fourteen treatments are in the books. Four more to go. Charlitude has hit the ball over the fence, and now it's just a trot around the bases.

Talk to you next week.

Rob

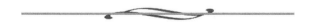

The "Why?" question is always difficult to answer in challenging situations. Often it takes days, weeks, months, or even years to reconcile. Once we realized that our relationship was better and we, both the two of us and our family, were happier than we had been previously without cancer, the "Why?" question was easier to contemplate. It became a less scary and empty question. We are supposed to live happy, satisfied lives, and cancer helped us do that.

The notion that having cancer in your life could somehow make you happier resonated with several people. We all experience things in life that we wish we didn't have to endure; however, so often on the other side of the event, we wouldn't change a thing. We are actually grateful for the trial. The theme I heard from others was "How can we experience all of the positives – inspiration, optimism and kindness – when things are going well? Why do we recognize and pursue these things after a trial? Why can't they stay on the forefront of our minds?"

The Saturday night before this update some good friends executed a perfect plan. They got a sitter at their house, all of our kids spent the night over there, and the four of us had an adult evening at our house. We had so much fun. Charlotte and I cooked dinner, they brought the wine, we set our dining room table with the fancy china, and we laughed together for hours. Charlotte and I then got to enjoy a slow, easy, quiet morning with coffee and the newspaper.

The gift-giving over the course of Charlotte's treatment needs some further attention. Unfortunately, no matter how hard I try to explain and document the incredible gifts of self that people extended our way, I cannot capture the emotion involved or how grateful we felt. Some of the biggest smiles on my face came from receiving inexpensive gifts. I enjoyed being blown away by people's thoughtfulness and ingenuity. "How did they come up with that?!?" It's great when friends position you to ask that question.

If you can't come up with a gift that is of yourself, give a gift card. Practical gifts like gift cards are always welcomed and are so useful. Every vendor in today's world can come up with a gift card. We received them for the meat market, for restaurants, the cleaners, and the liquor store. They don't have to be only for iTunes or a plain vanilla Visa card. Use a little creativity and get one from a local vendor that could use the business.

There were also a great number of anonymous gifts. Do you know how amazing it is to receive a gift with no strings attached? Gifts without even the small obligation of a thank-you note? We still to this day have no idea who gave us certain gifts, including the bright yellow Easter eggs with smiley faces painted on them that were in our front lawn Easter morning. The Easter Bunny has to be real.

Easter Sunday was crazy. My parents came into town, and we hosted brunch at our house. All of Charlotte's family came over, including her younger brother's in-laws. The house was a whirlwind of Easter eggs, chocolate, children, adults, entrées, desserts, pastel colors, baskets, bloody marys, and champagne.

As I work with Charlotte to raise our children, I often ponder, "Do I ignore that statement I just heard from the back seat, or do I address it?" Often both are correct, and it is a struggle to pick one. I have found, though, if there is an opportunity for growth by answering or not answering the statement or issue, silence is often the right choice. There is no chance, given the choice, we would have chosen cancer for Charlotte, but undoubtedly we are better people for having experienced cancer. I believe that many of our peers and friends would say the same thing.

We are also very grateful that the CA 125 test turned out to be such a good barometer for her cancer. There are people whose numbers don't track as consistently as Charlotte's, and that grieves Charlotte and me to our core. I wish there was a way to corral and squash the emotion that must come with test results that stay flat or move the other way. No one trying their best deserves that news. Please, Lord, give these patients peace.

It's not chemo. It's therapy.

CHAPTER 18
LET YOUR FRIENDS SEE YOUR PASSION

From: Rob Huthnance
Date: April 13, 2012 11:11:36 AM CDT
To: Rob Huthnance
Subject: 4/13/12 Charlotte Update

Dear Team Charlotte,

One of the byproducts of our situation is that I find myself very slow to return personal phone calls. I don't do it on purpose, and I don't really have an excuse. However, truth be told, it is taking me too long.

When I realized that I owed a friend a return call from last week, I sent him a text on Tuesday apologizing and promising to call. After hitting send, I scrolled through some previous texts we had shared and found this one that I sent to several people an hour after Charlotte's surgery on December 20.

"It was ovarian cancer, but they removed 100 percent of the disease. More details will follow this afternoon. The goal of the surgery was accomplished."

When I read this text from a few months before, I was drenched with visions and memories of that day. Then instantly, I couldn't believe how far we had come. As all these thoughts were racing through my head, we were driving to our son's baseball game, and we didn't have a care in the world. The windows were down, and we were all laughing as a family.

It's not chemo. It's therapy.

I was taken aback by how regimented and sterile the text was. I remember at the time thinking it was so positive. After all, step one was finished and successful. Now, a few months later, nothing in life seems worthy of being regimented and sterile.

So many of you, from lifelong friends to people I have never met in person, have been incredibly supportive of our family. One of the things I find amazing from this end of the keyboard is how much effort people have put into responding to the updates. Responses are never compulsory, and they are certainly not the goal of these updates. However, as people do respond, often we can tell that the person spent way more than sixty seconds crafting the email. On a couple of them, I would venture to guess that the author spent more time writing the response than I did on the actual update.

It hit me this week that the responses are never regimented or sterile. Each has its own individual passion, and I am grateful that such passion exists in people. So often we think we are supposed to act regimented, but it is such a release to reveal a passion that is somewhere inside us. The avenue by which passion is released doesn't matter. Just let it out.

I have two friends who bring passion to their golf attire. One looks like an Easter egg every time he steps up to the first tee, and the other wears only flat bill caps and looks like a 45-year-old Rickie Fowler. But I guarantee these two friends have more fun on the course than the guys wearing khaki shorts, a blue shirt, white shoes, and a curved white hat.

Charlotte's therapy session yesterday was scheduled to be a short one, but it took a few hours. Each week they draw a healthy-sized blood sample to check her blood counts. Routinely throughout this process, her blood counts have been above the acceptable levels. Yesterday the numbers came back quite low, so she had to receive special clearance from the doctor to receive the chemotherapy medicine.

This week was one of the smaller doses, and this weekend she is scheduled for shots to boost her blood counts. Knowing this, the doctor allowed the chemotherapy to be administered. The doctor has warned us since the beginning that in most cases patients' blood levels become too low to receive chemotherapy. When this happens, you have to delay the treatment for a time and perhaps receive a blood transfusion. We don't want delays or transfusions. She is determined to finish on schedule.

It's hard to believe, but fifteen rounds are in the books. Only three remain — one long session and two short ones.

On a personal note, I would like to thank each of you for your interest in these updates. You have allowed me to exploit a newfound aptitude, and I have developed a passion for putting my thoughts on paper. Thank you for helping me release it.

Talk to you next week.

Rob

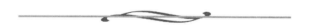

The Easter egg golfer has gotten some pretty good play around here. My favorite part about it is that my friend who dresses like an Easter egg is so proud of the grief he received. His email response to the update was simply, "And a very fancy Easter egg, at that." I'm confident that he is now more motivated than ever to look dapper on the course. We played as partners in a tournament a few weeks ago, and he did not disappoint, right down to his baby blue golf shoes.

Passion about something is so important. We all experience various levels of passion. It often comes and goes from people's lives, and you can always tell that someone is happier when passion is present in their lives. It doesn't matter what the passion is, either. It could be work, kids' sports, golf, dog training, cooking, fishing, reading, traveling, knifemaking, woodworking, playing guitar, or growing vegetables in your yard.

I have noticed a correlation between being passionate and celebrating, especially small victories. A person with sincere passion about something tends to celebrate small victories within that field. As I have reflected on these two items over the passing weeks, I've seen that people who aren't celebrating small victories regularly tend to not have passion for what they are doing. Whether it's work related, family related, or coaching a kids' sports team. The passionate coaches love helping the kids learn and excel, and they love giving a high five to the kid who always strikes out just because he foul-tipped the ball on his last at-bat. Other coaches often seem like they are on the sideline for other reasons.

Throughout my adult life, I have sought passion. However, it took my wife's developing cancer for me to recognize that. I enjoy work, love my family, laugh with my friends, but passion still seemed elusive. I am enthusiastic about 99 percent of my activities and engagements, but enthusiasm is different from passion. The thesaurus lists these words as synonyms, but the dictionary defines them differently. Enthusiasm is excited interest, and passion is intense emotion. We can always muster up excited interest, but it's that intense emotion that we all crave. Intense emotion is what sets off the fireworks inside us and wills us to do more.

If Charlotte wasn't the passionate person that she is, there is no way she would have received treatment this week. It would have been too easy for the nurse to whisper, "It's no big deal. Let's wait a couple days and try again." No one was about to say this to her. For months now, Charlotte has made the entire staff feel great about their jobs and duties, and they were going to return the favor by helping and allowing her to charge forward.

CHAPTER 19
ALWAYS SADDLE YOUR OWN HORSE

From: Rob Huthnance
Date: April 20, 2012 10:59:48 AM CDT
To: Rob Huthnance
Subject: 4/20/12 Charlotte Update

Dear Team Charlotte,

Charlotte attended Camp Waldemar every summer as a child. She was the camper every parent wants their child to be. She loved every minute, was never homesick, was friends with everyone, and won many awards. Last weekend Camp Waldemar hosted family camp. We drove the six hours to Hunt, Texas, with the children and had a great time. The Texas Hill Country is a special place, and the setting at Waldemar is unparalleled.

From the moment we drove through the front gate, Charlotte was in her element. The owners and staff were all awaiting her arrival and were very excited to see her. Several of her camp peers were also there for the weekend. The girls, now women, relived old memories, laughed until their sides hurt, and discussed how they hoped their girls would one day have the same experiences.

Charlotte's favorite activity was horseback riding. The woman who taught horseback riding taught thousands of girls over the years, and finally retired when she passed away at the age of 101.

The most lasting lesson each of the girls learned from her was her mandate to "always saddle your own horse." This lesson transcends well beyond horseback riding. Connie Reeves was the teacher's name, and she is enshrined in the Texas Cowgirl Hall of Fame.

It's my opinion that Camp Waldemar was integral in forming the basis for Charlitude.

You remember in college, right before you turned twenty-one, trying to get into the best college bar? You knew you could control yourself, you knew it was fun inside, and at that very moment there was nothing more important in the world than getting through the doors. Then, at the last second, the bouncer wouldn't let you in.

You walked away feeling dejected, mad, and frustrated. After a few minutes, you knew things were going to be fine, but you were still bitter that you couldn't party with everyone else. Yesterday, we felt exactly that feeling.

When we arrived at the doctor's office, we went through the normal routine of checking in and having blood drawn. By now Charlotte is best friends with everyone who works there, and the women at the front desk couldn't stop talking about how cute her top was. Then the nurse who weighed her and took her blood pressure asked her if she drove a white Suburban. Charlotte said yes, and everyone laughed, because the nurse had seen a white Suburban in the parking lot with smiley face stickers on it and suspected it was Charlotte's.

As is customary before each of the long chemotherapy sessions, we have an appointment with the oncologist to discuss overall health, side effects, the current state of affairs, future issues, and potential concerns.

All of that part of the conversation went well. Then he told us about her current blood levels. Her white blood cell count was too low for chemotherapy. By no means is this devastating or cause for concern, but it was a big blow. We are so close to being finished.

We already knew everything the doctor told us. Blood levels fall during chemotherapy, she had done extremely well to make it this far without any sort of delay, and by living her normal lifestyle, the white blood cells will increase in a few days. Time is the only remedy. It's just a bummer and nothing else.

I have shared the story about the delay with chemotherapy on one condition — no one gets to call and say how sorry they are that she didn't get to have therapy yesterday. Neither sympathy nor empathy is allowed within the walls of Charlitude. As you all know by now, Charlitude focuses only on the positive. Yesterday's occurrence was not a bad thing. We are grateful that the doctor's have the ability to test blood levels and know when to slow down.

Last night a friend put it well and said that the flight was not cancelled. We are simply in a weather delay. And just like in college, Charlotte will get to go to the party next week, and a couple of months from now no one will remember the party she missed.

Feel free to reach out to her if you have a good joke or a funny story. Laughter is always welcome and is a key component to Charlitude.

We are expecting a nice low-key weekend, and we are expecting her bone marrow to do its job and produce a herd of white blood cells. Charlotte's spirit will do its part. We need her body to do the rest. After flourishing throughout this ordeal, I think it goes without saying that Miss Connie would be proud of how well Charlotte saddles her own horse.

Talk to you next week.

Rob

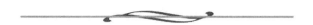

Charlotte can't wait for the girls to go to camp. So much so that family camp at Waldemar has been on the calendar for a year, and our older daughter C.C. still has two more summers before she can attend. Charlotte and I were both summer campers as children, and we want our children to experience camp life. Summer camp is one of the most empowering events a child can experience. I remember vividly the feeling of freedom and maturing that comes with summer camp. Our son has gone the last three summers to camp. Each year when we pick him up, from the first moment we lay eyes on him, we can see that his confidence and maturity have elevated.

Charlotte has dozens if not hundreds of connections to people who went to Camp Waldemar. I can't tell you how often someone asks, "Do you know so-and-so?" only to hear her say, "Sure, we went to camp together." If you were five years on either side of Charlotte's age at camp, she remembers you.

Even with the recent low blood counts, we had been cruising through chemotherapy so smoothly that we were stunned by this week's setback. Of course we always knew a delay was possible, if not probable, but we were so close to the end that we didn't believe it was going to happen to us. Charlotte's blood counts stayed elevated on their own for such a long time, and then her bone marrow responded so well to the shots that we thought we were home free. Thirty minutes after we left the doctor's office we were fine, but those thirty minutes were not very fun. A friend had accompanied us this week, and she was certainly surprised to see both of us walk back into the waiting room carrying all of Charlotte's magazines, blankets, and other gear that traveled to therapy with her. It was nice having another person in the car with us for the ride home. She was able to clear some of the intense air for us.

I was very hesitant about sharing this news about the delay because I could see so many people with good intentions reaching out to Charlotte only to say how sorry they were. This type of sympathy has never set well with her, and the delay was the perfect set-up. However, everyone honored my request to not bombard her with sympathy. We went on about our day and looked forward to the weekend.

I have heard Miss Connie's mantra, "Always saddle your own horse," so many times because it fits so many situations. I knew from the moment I started typing the update that I would end it with that line. I was so glad I could make it fit.

CHAPTER 20
YOU GET TO DO THINGS LIKE THIS ONLY ONCE

From: Rob Huthnance
Date: April 27, 2012 11:04:50 AM CDT
To: Rob Huthnance
Subject: 4/27/12 Charlotte Update

Dear Team Charlotte,

Last weekend the alumni association at Charlotte's high school held a ceremony to induct four teachers into the school's hall of fame. One of the teachers taught Charlotte's little brother as well as our two older children. Over the years, she and Charlotte have been friends and confidants, and she asked Charlotte to present her at the ceremony. Charlotte was touched by the offer and was happy to do it.

Two hundred people attended the event. Charlotte prepared well for her speech and gave an excellent delivery. I have seen her speak in public many times, and I believe this was her best presentation. The teacher gave thirty-three years for that one evening, and I'm glad Charlotte gave her her best.

The teacher has a wonderful later-in-life love story, and her new fiancé approached Charlotte after the speeches were finished. He thanked her for doing a good job, and then said, "You get to do things like this only once." Meaning there is only one induction into a hall of fame. Even if it does not go as planned, there is no mulligan, no do-over for a night like this.

It's not chemo. It's therapy.

I love that line. "You get to do things like this only once." It really got my attention when I heard it. There are so many things in life that really happen only once, and unfortunately, we often don't take full advantage of that one time. I intend to better recognize these one-time events and genuinely pause and take notice as they are happening.

After the party was finished, someone had the great idea to convince the entertainment (guy and his guitar) that playing for us at our house was the right thing to do. Next thing you know, four couples and our new friend were on our back porch holding Styrofoam cups and singing all the words we could remember to favorite songs. I have been with musicians playing music late at night a time or two in the past, but no one else has the talent we heard that night. He didn't miss a note or fumble a string, and he played every song requested by "the crowd." It was big fun; however, it took our Saturday night way too far into Sunday morning.

Things like that happen only once. We will more than likely listen to a guy and his guitar on our back porch again, but odds are it won't be our newest friend and the crowd will be different.

By the way, the musician didn't have one sticker on his guitar case. He never has, and he has been playing for twenty years. True to Charlitude, he left our house after voluntarily adding a yellow smiley face sticker to his black guitar case.

After the false start at the doctor's office last week, we rescheduled the appointment for Monday morning. Our expectations were high, but secretly we were hoping that our lack of sleep over the weekend didn't jeopardize her blood counts. The machine they use for blood tests provided a result that was right on the cut line.

For patients who don't show up wearing all things smiley face, I am certain the nurses would have simply said, "Sorry, let's try again in a couple of days."

However, in an effort to grant Charlotte's wish of putting therapy in the rearview mirror, the technician (and friend by now) examined the sample manually under a microscope. This extra effort determined that her white blood cell count was high enough to proceed. One stick of the needle and a couple hours later the last long session was behind her.

Last year a friend from Dallas moved to Kentucky. There she happened to become friends with one of Charlotte's good friends from college. A month ago they bought plane tickets to come to Dallas to attend a therapy session with Charlotte. Little did they know when they bought the tickets that Charlotte's schedule would be rearranged.

Consequently, during their quick visit in Dallas, the only responsibility they had was to have fun. What a blessing last week's low blood count turned out to be. The old friends didn't have to waste any of their precious time together sitting in the infusion suite. I had to take a quick overnight trip on Wednesday, and I am very grateful that they were at our house to be with Charlotte.

Monday is the new day for therapy. Two short sessions remain.

Chemotherapy is something we want to do only once. We have paused and taken notice all along the way.

Talk to you next week.

Rob

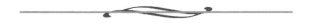

When I heard "you get to do things like this only once," I loved it and knew it would make the update in some form. I am very fond of experiences that can happen only once. They provide excellent memories. Charlotte loves to take photographs, and I honestly don't because too often I feel like photos interrupt the flow of the moment. I do enjoy looking at photos years after the actual event, but they rarely match the scene that I have in my mind's eye. When Charlotte and I were married, we discussed videotaping our rehearsal dinner. Given my derelict group of friends, I was nervous about having the speeches recorded and forever saved. I also didn't want to video the dinner because I wanted people, including myself, to not feel the need to perform for the camera. I knew that the night would be a great memory, and there are some things that are just better left as that … a memory.

This teacher Hall of Fame night was another thing for Charlotte to look forward to. It had been on the calendar for several weeks, and Charlotte had to prepare a speech. This is not something she does every day so it took a little effort to get it right. Focusing on the speech was a great distraction from the mundane cancer stuff.

Charlotte and I have a hard time saying no to a good time. I've never understood how people can consistently be the first ones to leave a party or be the first ones to go to bed while on a group vacation. I'm always one of the last people standing because I'm afraid I will miss out on something. Don't let her fool you, Charlotte has been known to stay up even later than I on occasion. What if someone tells a funny story or dances with a lampshade on his head or trips in front of everyone? I know I'm rolling the dice on this because I could easily be the one everyone laughs at, but it's worth the gamble to stay up late just to see what crazy antics might take place.

When the opportunity window cracked slightly and there was an opportunity for the musician to come over to our house, we stood behind him and shoved him through the window. I can't explain it, but there is nothing more fun than listening to live music in an intimate setting, especially when the musician is this good. He was like a human jukebox. What a great memory, even though we paid for it the next day.

What are the odds that a friend of ours from Dallas moves to a town in Kentucky with 10,000 people in it and the first person she meets is one of Charlotte's roommates from college? That's exactly what happened. Knowing therapy was scheduled on Thursdays, the two new friends picked a Thursday – weeks in advance – and booked their trip around it. However, when the time came, and we experienced the delay, the whole schedule and tune of the trip changed – for the better.

We had the best time with our friends from Kentucky. The only thing on the agenda was fun, and that was such a gift. Charlotte and her girlfriends took full advantage of their time together. They had long lunches, went shopping, laughed, reminisced, stayed up late, stayed in their pajamas well into the morning, and just acted silly, like good friends who hadn't seen each other in a while.

Given the timing of the delay and then the joy of being with friends, this situation clearly felt like the Lord was giving us one of those "I told you not to worry" lessons. You can attach a myriad of phrases to the therapy delay, including it was part of the plan, I told you so, I know what I'm doing, trust me, or do your job and I'll do mine. We could hear the man upstairs saying all of these things to us. All we could say was "Okay, okay – and thank you!"

CHAPTER 21
OH MY GOODNESS, IT'S THE FINISH LINE!

From: Rob Huthnance
Date: May 4, 2012 10:44:18 AM CDT
To: Rob Huthnance
Subject: 5/4/12 Charlotte Update

Dear Team Charlotte,

We can see the finish line, and no one is in front of us …

After seventeen chemotherapy sessions, this is how we feel. I'm not much of a runner. In fact, I exercise only to stay alive another day and to be able to swing a golf club marginally more consistently. However, I can imagine how it must feel to win a long, grueling race. Exhaustion, elation, relief, restoration, renewal, fatigue, ecstasy, and liberation are all words that come to mind.

This past weekend we were able to get some rest. Friday night our son had a baseball game, and Saturday night we had some friends over for home-smoked barbecue while the kids swam in the pool. The sermon at church on Sunday was great, and that afternoon Thompson and I had a heated golf match with another father/son team. Charlotte, meanwhile, took the girls to the Barnyard Bash in the church parking lot.

Before school on Monday morning, we followed our ritual of breaking the links in the paper chain made for this journey. It was very encouraging to see the single lonely link left on the mantel above the fireplace.

It's not chemo. It's therapy.

A friend took Charlotte to her therapy session later Monday morning. Her blood counts were low; however, since it was a short session, they allowed her to proceed. Charlotte did have to promise to stay away from "germy" places for a few days. It was a one-stick event, and they were out of there in no time. Charlotte was able to take her customary nap thanks to the pre-game Benadryl.

The schedule for next week is as follows: Monday morning Charlotte has her final therapy session. Shortly after lunch she gets to go through the door on the left side of the waiting room at the oncologist's office (instead of the right side) for the first time. Here she will get to drink "the stuff" and have a full-body CT scan. She meets with the doctor Thursday morning to discuss her results and final resolutions. Then, celebrate like never before!

For some reason the CT scan on Monday feels a little intimidating. We are expecting perfection, and there is no reason to expect otherwise. After everything we have been through, this should be easy. They are taking pictures of her insides only to confirm that the surgery and chemotherapy accomplished their missions. Yet waiting for the results has similarities to the anxious feeling of waiting for a child to be born. You know that everyone has done their job — the good Lord, doctors, nurses, technicians, Charlotte, family, friends, even strangers — nothing should go wrong. However, hearing the word "Congratulations" has never been so anticipated or desired.

There are so many people witnessing this journey with us. Please put Monday after lunch on your calendar. Regarding the CT scan, once again, we are asking for everyone's thoughts and prayers.

We are so close. All week our friends have been so excited for us. Through their enthusiasm and excitement, I swear you can hear the roar of the crowd as we approach the finish line. The man with the stopwatch has his finger on the button. He is ready to press it and yell "Time!"

Talk to you next week.

Rob

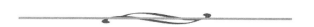

The 17th and penultimate therapy session felt very tangible. But after so many sessions, what's one more? And it was a short one at that.

Seventeen of the eighteen links in the paper chain were colorful. The final and only remaining link was white. The color white represented the light at the end of the tunnel. It's easy to see the difference in the length of the chain when a number of links have been removed. There is a marked difference between fourteen links and six links, but the difference in length is hard to distinguish from week to week, with just one link being removed at a time. There is not a lot of difference between twelve links and eleven links. However, with only one link remaining, and a white link at that, you knew the end was near.

We all have lived for that distant day in the future. It's the day that marks the culmination of hard work and stamina. Whether it is a graduation, big payday, wedding or birth, we have all experienced the excitement of being so close to that one day. You didn't think the day would ever arrive, but lo and behold, you can now count the hours. It's so exciting.

However, with cancer, there is always this cloud hanging over your head. You constantly want to look over your shoulder. Is this really the last day? Is her body strong enough to hold cancer at bay? Throughout this journey we have learned it's okay to look over your shoulder from time to time. It's okay to be smart about certain decisions that could affect your health. Just don't get bogged down and let these thoughts run your life. There's too much living to do.

The result of the CT scan was our focus. We didn't talk about it a lot, but we were both anxious. We knew how important that picture was. We had been through so much and had tried so hard physically, mentally, and spiritually. We didn't want to be undermined by a picture. However, just thinking about those results caused extremely conflicting emotions. One thought brought sheer exuberance, and the other brought terrible apprehension. We know that our psyche and attitudes are better when we concern ourselves only with what we know, but it was hard to not think about the unknowns of the CT scan.

Frankly, by the time Monday came around, I had forgotten that I had requested thoughts and prayers for that day's doctor's appointment. I was reminded at around 2 p.m. when I received an email from a nice guy who really is more of an acquaintance than a friend. His email noted that we had been on his calendar and he was praying that we were celebrating like crazy. Wow, thank you.

The girlfriend who accompanied Charlotte to therapy this week deserves more credit than I can give. She performed none of the examples of help I describe throughout the book, yet during Charlotte's entire journey, this girlfriend never left Charlotte's side. I wish I could provide some specific examples of her helpfulness, but I can't. There are just too many and none of them is dramatic. She simply did all the little things that no one else offered to do, and these were often the things with which Charlotte needed the most help. She deserves more than this paragraph, but her acts were never about chasing status or wanting a pat on the back. All we can really say is "Thank you."

There were several great responses to this week's update, but my favorite was from a friend in California. It simply read, "Can you hear us roaring?"

It's not chemo. It's therapy.

CHAPTER 22
I GENUINELY TRIED MY BEST

From: Rob Huthnance
Date: May 11, 2012 10:59:02 AM CDT
To: Rob Huthnance
Subject: 5/11/12 Charlotte Update

Since the days each of my three children were born, while only in my mind and never on paper, I have been "writing" each of their wedding rehearsal dinner speeches.

I don't sleep through the night very often, and over the years I have enjoyed lying awake thinking about what I will say. For the old friends who attended my rehearsal dinner and will be at one or all of my children's, I promise the speeches will be shorter than the one I gave on May 8, 1998.

Each child has a different personality; therefore, each speech has to be different. Each crowd will have a different feel, and I expect the surroundings and venues will be different as well. I love thinking about this.

I get emotional 99 percent of the time when the thoughts enter my mind, and I still have years to go.

In the same manner that I have been thinking about what I might say at my children's rehearsal dinners, I have thought about this update. It is the final one.

Over the last several months, I have contemplated different ways of imparting the wisdom we have gained from this experience. I kept notes along the way just for this update. However, now that the time is here, I don't know what else I can say to all of you.

It's not chemo. It's therapy.

So this update is just for Charlotte, but joyfully, I am including all of you who have been so supportive.

Dear Charlotte,

From the moment we learned of your probable diagnosis, I have experienced anxiety, apprehension, angst, uncertainty, insecurity, courage, and joy, but I was never scared. As the doctor told us yesterday, I always knew your cancer would be in full remission after this process. Without being clairvoyant, I also "knew" that at some point the doctor's head nurse would say how she had been doing her job for years and she had never seen anyone handle this like you. Those words came on Monday – therapy's final day.

I have been told that as you get older you start to think of your marriage in terms of years. Some years were good years, and some years were not as good. Even though we have been married for only fourteen years, I can comprehend this fact. The year 2007 was an incredible year for us. Candidly, 2011 was not. The stress in our marriage was higher than it had ever been, and then you got sick. Suddenly the self-imposed stress of 2011 seemed like tiddlywinks.

Oddly, within a couple of weeks of your diagnosis, your cancer made us better – a lot better. I will gladly accept my share of the blame, and I'm sorry you had to go through this ordeal. However, I am so grateful you did. Thank you.

I am grateful that you were given the opportunity to show the world that people can be happy with cancer in their lives. I am grateful that because of your effort people will have a positive attitude from the first minute they receive their diagnosis. I am grateful that our children never missed a beat. And I am grateful that we want to be better.

I was always more anxious than you about your being bald. No matter where we were when you got a hot flash and took off your scarf, I held my breath. I hope you never noticed. I genuinely tried my best. While you were getting your necessary rest, I was out of my comfort zone with duties around the house. Making breakfast and getting the children ready for school each day provided more challenges than I had ever imagined. I hope you didn't hear us scrambling downstairs. I genuinely tried my best. Every time friends and strangers put their hands on your shoulders to promote your healing, I held back my emotions. I wanted to be strong because I knew when the person walked away, you would melt and would need additional strength. I hope I was strong enough. I genuinely tried my best.

The children are convinced cancer is beatable; nevertheless, they truly believe every family will fight this fight at some point. I hope they are wrong about that. I don't know when Thompson, C.C. and Georgeann will finally realize what this family has endured, but I suspect it will be when they have children the ages of nine, seven, and five.

I also don't know why we were chosen to experience so much at what seems like such an early age. Our whole lives, both of us always wanted to play with the older kids. So many of our best friends are several years older than we are, and yet we now have more experience than most of them. Before cancer, the thought of sharing our experiences with others was petrifying. Now it's exhilarating. I can't wait to help others get through similar situations.

Charlitude and your tenacity and powerful spirit will serve as an example to many, many people. Thousands of people have followed your journey. Hundreds of these people will be diagnosed with cancer in their lifetimes. Your efforts and example will make their battle easier.

Both the Old and New Testaments proclaim, "You reap what you sow." Throughout this experience, your harvest has been more bountiful than ever imagined. Your entire life you have been an incredible friend to others. Often to my frustration, you willingly gave your time and resources to friends in need. Your friends have returned everything to you tenfold, and through all of these blessings, you were able to "smile your way through it."

Sometime around the year 2028, I can't wait to watch your smiling face as I give my first rehearsal dinner speech for one our three beloved children.

I love you. Congratulations … Cheers … and Thank You.

Rob

P.S. Many of you have encouraged me to keep writing after this chapter is finished. Thank you for the kind words. I plan to do so. I don't know what shape this will take, but I will find an avenue. I also would like to reserve the right to reach out to everyone on this list from time to time. I expect I will witness something encouraging, and I know I will want to share it.

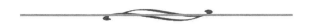

I thought about this update for weeks, and I even found myself daydreaming about it. I didn't know which direction it would take, but I could see it on the horizon. We knew there were eighteen chemotherapy sessions, so there was an impending end to the updates once we were finished with treatment. The more I thought about it, the less I felt like a real estate developer and the more I felt like a writer. After enduring such an ordeal and having to carry such a heavy load, that feeling of stepping outside my comfort zone and the change of pace were both comforting and exciting.

I had several guy friends, privately through email and sometimes in person, tell me how they got emotional and actually teared up while reading one or more updates. I took this as a challenge and wanted to strike that nerve with this final update. As I tried to connect with people's emotions, I wanted them to feel just what I was feeling. While it is impossible to feel the emotion that comes with cancer without the actual cancer experience, every married person has a bond and emotional connection, and I wanted to associate my cancer experience with the feelings you have only for your spouse.

One evening in early April, I sat down with my laptop and just started writing this update. The rehearsal dinner comments just flowed out of my fingers. Once those were on paper, the "Letter to Charlotte" idea came to mind. I was all by myself, and I couldn't keep it together. I was a mess. I was so pleased yet overwhelmed with the concept that I struggled to write the content. I didn't know yet what I would write, but I wanted to say things to her directly that I couldn't say in a regular update. In the coming weeks, every time I added a line or two, I fell apart. I toiled with the final update off and on for weeks, and I tweaked words and phrases right up to the moment I clicked send.

I lived so closely to each week's update. I knew them backward and forward, and I had my own sentimental connection with each one. This weekly bond came from thinking through all the information and the corresponding emotions and tying the two together. Because of these updates, every Friday I enjoyed a sense of accomplishment, and thankfully, my words helped Charlotte gain vigor and inspiration to press forward. The updates also seemed to inspire the community to do more good.

I'm not sure whether it was that I thought I would lose some of my identity now that the weekly updates would no longer be necessary, or whether it was that I had put so much of my soul into this final update, but after I clicked send, I could hardly catch my breath. Because I had thought about the last update for so long, I felt closer to this final one than any of the others. I was alone in my office, and my chest tightened up so badly that I was concerned about a heart attack. Since I had a strong pulse, I concluded that I was having some sort of anxiety attack, something I had never experienced before. I relaxed on the couch in my office until I could finally breathe normally again. It took longer than I would have liked.

All spring after people read each update, they responded via email. I never knew who would respond or what they would say. It was always random, too. Each update affected people differently, meaning there was no consistent pattern to those who responded. I suspect people would reply only if something I'd written struck a nerve somewhere, and the immediate responses were always by email. After this final email, though, my phone rang. I couldn't hide behind my computer. On the phone, I had to address questions straight on. This was a little unnerving, but proved helpful for both ends of the phone line.

During this experience and every day since, I have thought a lot about my children. Will this end up being a brief recollection from their childhood, or will this be a defining moment in their lives? Will they be able to help the next kid in their class who encounters cancer in their family? As badly as I want this memory and all that they witnessed to simply fade away, they each have a personality that can handle the added responsibility. Surely the Lord can use them to help other children, and surely they can help without bogging down in their own challenging memories.

I know for a fact that during my marriage to Charlotte she has always gone overboard to help an acquaintance in need, and I'm reasonably certain she was doing this for years before I met her. By way of example, oftentimes during her treatment when I arrived home from work, she would be in the kitchen cooking. At first glance this seemed very normal. The kids were running around the house being kids, and she was simply cooking dinner. However, she was cooking dinner for another family.

Once I realized what was going on, I would ask whom she was cooking for, and often she would have to explain how we were connected to the people receiving dinner. To me, she was just adding stress to her life. To her, she was doing what she was put here to do.

The final drive to the doctor's office was very quiet. It was just the two of us. No friends were there to break the tension. We knew in our bones that she was well, but still we were nervous.

It's hard to explain or describe the anxiety associated with anticipating this appointment. I can recall many times in life that I thought were life-and-death moments – waiting for the phone call from the coach about making the majors in Little League, asking a girl to the eighth-grade dance, or opening my acceptance letter from the University of Texas. What a wimp I was for thinking those events were vital to survival. The results of those events were nothing compared with living my life without my wife.

When we met with the doctor, he was all business, which was fine. We talked about multiple side effects, things to look out for, and expectations for the future. At the end of our conversation, he finally cracked a big smile, stood up, and said "Congratulations!"

Oh, how I love that word.

We can't thank our community enough for grabbing us around the neck and pulling us along. Everyone we know played a part in our success. Thank you.

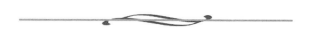

~ Postscript ~

The email updates started as a way to keep friends and family abreast of Charlotte's condition. Along the way they morphed into a way for my family to thank those who helped us, a way to provide a little humor and insight, and a means of giving examples of how people can help each other within a community.

In this spirit of helping others, the idea for this book presented itself. The purpose of this book is not only to use our story and experiences to help patients and caregivers going through challenging times, but also to provide some easy, yet meaningful, ideas for supporters, those who are in a position to help people in need.

After living through cancer on a daily basis for months, I can intimately understand and comprehend what Paul was telling us in his letter to the Corinthians.

2 Corinthians 1:3-4
New International Version (NIV)

Praise be to the God and Father of our Lord Jesus
Christ, the Father of compassion and the God of all
comfort, who comforts us in all our troubles, so that
we can comfort those in any trouble with the comfort
we ourselves receive from God.

We positively received comfort from the Lord, but numerous friends and strangers who had suffered previous troubles also comforted us. It is now our turn to return the favor and pay it forward.

When someone in your community is in need, please ponder about what you can offer them. Each of us is uniquely talented, and our friends know what those talents are. Donate your talents and not something out of obligation. If you can't boil water, don't offer to cook someone dinner. Run errands, organize medical bills, wash a car, pull weeds and plant flowers, run the carpool, or write a heartfelt note. Gifts of self are always more appreciated by the recipient and are always more fun to give.

AUTHOR'S NOTE

I need to share a story about a friend whose contribution to our family's success is immeasurable. We live across the street from Alison and Mike Malone. On December 21, 2009, their little boy Michael was diagnosed with neuroblastoma, a rare form of cancer found in children. About 650 cases are diagnosed annually in the United States. The easiest way to describe this cancer is as a young child grows, the cells in the spinal cord do not know how to "die." Instead, the cells form cancerous tumors. Michael was 4½ when he was diagnosed.

Because of him and his battle, our children had a significant understanding of cancer. They lived it with him and through him on a daily basis. They visited him in the hospital, they played together when he felt well enough, and they watched him fight miraculously. He allowed us to discuss and explain cancer in a way that would have been impossible had he not been in our lives.

After 2½ years, on June 23, 2012, Michael's body succumbed to cancer.

Michael had wisdom well beyond his years. He was brilliantly smart, communicated effectively, and had a wonderful attitude. We are very grateful for the time we were given with Michael, and we are so blessed that he helped all of us approach cancer in a positive way. To help others fight cancer, please consider Wipe Out Kids Cancer (wokc.org).

Thank you Alison and Mike for raising your son as you did.

And thank you, Michael.

ACKNOWLEDGMENTS

The encouragement I have received to see this project through has been remarkable and unparalleled compared with any other project I have embarked upon in my life. It took longer than I ever contemplated, but I joyfully drove the sled with my legs pumping the whole time. All the while, our friends acted as coaches cheering me on.

I am forever grateful for the relentless support, and I am so indebted to all for inspiring me to pursue this newfound passion.

I would like to give special appreciation to Charlotte, who showed all of us the power of a positive attitude. I am so blessed that our children not only took everything in stride, but also excelled through a difficult time.

To Doctors Oh, Nockleberg, and Shires for their wisdom, calmness, and amazing abilities.

Thank you to the lady in the waiting room while Charlotte endured her first CT scan, and to Charlotte's family, my family, the Hyer moms, all our friends throughout our community, Ole Miss friends, Texas friends, Therapy friends, champagne celebrations, the friends who annihilated cancer before us, complete strangers who sought us out, my mother's prayer team,

Amy Bowling, Kelly Andersson, the nurses in the infusion suite at Texas Oncology in Plano, the Mary Crowley Cancer Research Center – and of course, the words *Thank You*.

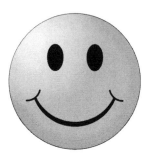

ABOUT THE AUTHOR

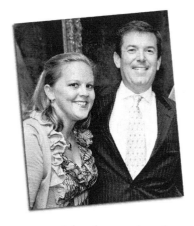

Rob Huthnance is a native Texan, attended the University of Texas and lives with his family in Dallas.

He has spent his entire career in developing commercial real estate, but through his wife's journey with ovarian cancer, he has found a passion for writing and helping others in need.

Rob Huthnance has a blog online:
itsnotchemo.com